The Herbal
Health and Beauty
Book

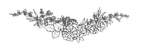

The Herbal Health and Beauty Book

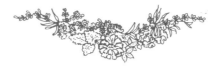

Hilary Boddie

PHOTOGRAPHS BY GIDEON HART
ILLUSTRATED BY KATHY LAMBERT

O P T I M A

An OPTIMA Book

First published in Great Britain by
Optima in 1994

ISBN 0 356 21030 8

Typeset by Solidus (Bristol) Limited
Printed and bound in Great Britain by
BPC Hazell Books Ltd
A member of
The British Printing Company Ltd

Optima
A Division of
Little, Brown and Company (UK) Limited
Brettenham House
Lancaster Place
London WC2E 7EN

Contents

Acknowledgements

I would like to express my wholehearted thanks to the following for all their help and hard work: Beverley D'Silva, with whom I worked out the original concept for the book; Mr Hein Zeylstra, Director of the School of Phytotherapy (Herbal Medicine) for his expert guidance; to Gideon Hart for the excellent photographs; to Rosemary Titterington of Iden Croft Herbs for the superb plants; to Kathy Lambert for her wonderful illustrations; Helen Ambrosen, Arts and Sciences Director for Cosmetics To Go, for her help in developing the beauty recipes; plus formulations and technical advice from Montagne Jeunesse, a leading ethical toiletries company, whose products are formulated by herbalists.

Author's note

The advice contained in this book is general and not specific to individuals and their particular circumstances. Any plant substance can cause an allergic reaction and any application of the techniques, ideas and suggestions in this book is at the reader's sole discretion and risk. The author and publisher of this book cannot be held responsible for any adverse reaction caused through the mistaken identity of herbs or the inappropriate use of any herbal preparation.

The techniques, suggestions and ideas in this book are not intended as a substitute for medical advice. If you are in any doubt about treating yourself, relatives or friends, consult a qualified practitioner or doctor. Even the mildest symptoms may have a serious origin.

Introduction

There is nothing new in harnessing the power of plants to improve health and appearance. Herbal remedies and cosmetics have been used to great effect throughout history, and as concern grows about both the side effects of many of today's synthetic drugs and the growing list of additives, preservatives and colourants incorporated in modern cosmetics, more and more people are now looking for more natural and totally safe alternatives that they can use and enjoy.

This book is intended as a comprehensive and straight-forward guide to the use of the healing and therapeutic properties of plants to benefit the body. Herbs are not only inexpensive and easy to obtain or grow, but they are simple to use and a lot of fun too. There's a certain magic in a whole herb. Each one contains a unique blend of active principles and other ingredients to which the living body is highly receptive.

Harnessing these beneficial properties, through making your own herbal preparations, will not only give you peace of mind that what you are using is safe, natural and effective, but it will also afford you greater control over your own health and general well-being. Get to know herbs – they can be great friends!

The secret life of plants

As well as being a source of natural living beauty and part of the vegetation that characterises our country-side, plants – and in particular herbs – have long since played an altogether more practical role in society. For they are also a source of valuable active constituents known to have a healing and beneficial effect on the body. And for thousands of years these unique plant properties have been used in the treatment and prevention of illness and for enhancing the body by many civilisations throughout the world. From ancient Egypt to the classical world of Rome and Greece, from Persia to India, China and Russia, herbs at one time were the basis of all medicines and cosmetics.

The Chinese have a very strong tradition of using herbal remedies. The Pen-ts'ao or *Canon of Herbs*, compiled over 5000 years ago by Emperor Wen Shen-Nung, included 252 plant descriptions and notes on their effects on the body. It was the first authoritative chronicle of its kind in Chinese history. These ancient texts are still studied and followed by many practitioners in China today. According to the traditional system of Chinese medicine, a physician does not look for a single cause of a disease or symptom but for imbalances or patterns of disharmony within the person as a whole. And today, herbs – in conjunction with other therapies such as acupuncture and massage – are still employed to help correct such imbalances.

The ancient Egyptians were also great users of herbs. The Ebers Papyrus written around 1500BC lists over 700 herbal remedies, many of which are still in use today. The Egyptians also imported large quantities of fragrant gums, resins, roots and barks from northern India and southern Arabia for cosmetic use and applied dried henna leaves to give their cheeks a healthy, rosy glow and to colour the hair. When the Pharaoh Tutankhamun was buried, the contents of his tomb included a bottle of perfumed oil which was still found to be potent some 3000 years later.

Records discovered by archaeologists prove that nations such as Persia, India and the Aztecs of South America possessed knowledge of the medicinal and cosmetic use of plants thousands of years before the birth of Christ. The ancient Indian Ayurvedic system of medicine, like traditional Chinese medicine, sees illness in terms of imbalance, and uses herbs and dietary controls to restore the balance. The earliest Ayurvedic texts and Sumerian herbals both date from around 2500BC and tablets discovered from the library of the King of Assyria mention some 250 plant medicines. It was also common practice for Assyrian women to whiten their face with herbal powders to give their skin a delicate smoothness.

The ancient Greeks ascribed a divine origin to flowers and leaves and used them for both sweet-smelling perfumes as well as herbal remedies. It was believed that if one of the gods were to honour anyone with a visit, they would leave behind a sweet scent as a token of their divinity. Thus the Greeks began to use perfumes made from aromatic plants and spices such as myrrh, frankincense and cinnamon, on a large scale.

The Greek physician Hippocrates, known as the 'father of medicine', who was responsible for developing the first scientific system of medicine, refers to 300 medicinal plants in his writings. He divided all plants and foods into four categories – hot, cold, damp and dry – and maintained that good health was achieved through keeping a balance between them.

Other notable physicians of the classical world, namely the Roman writer Pliny (the most quoted author from ancient Rome), Theophrastus (often described as the 'father of botany'), Dioscorides and Galen all described the use of herbal remedies in their various writings on medical botany, many of which were still being quoted and studied in the seventeenth century. Similarly, the practice of using herbal cosmetics was continued and greatly expanded by the Romans. In particular they used St John's wort, myrtle and walnut to darken the hair, myrtle and juniper berries to treat baldness, whilst fragrant plants were macerated in grease and rubbed into the hair to prevent it falling out. They also took therapeutic baths scented with bay and rosemary leaves.

After the fall of the Roman Empire in the fifth century AD, in the so-called Dark Ages, many of the herbal traditions were neglected and it was monks who kept the interest in herbs and their healing potential alive. Caring for the sick was thought of as an important Christian duty and monks, who used herbal remedies, became the first general physicians in their local communities. Also, as they travelled from one monastery to another, valuable information regarding the different healing properties contained within the herbs was passed on and shared, and it was behind monastic walls that the first formal herb gardens were established. By the end of the seventeenth century, physic gardens had been laid out throughout Europe. The Chelsea Physic Garden in London was founded by the

Worshipful Society of Apothecaries in 1673 and can still be found on the same site today.

Herbs were also used for their hair colouring properties and plants such as turmeric, rhubarb and the bark of the bearberry tree were all recommended for 'a most fair and beautiful colour'. However, with the advent of printing in the fifteenth century, it was the medicinal rather than the cosmetic value of herbs that rose to prominence in the West. The medicinal herbal remedies of antiquity became more accessible in the form of printed textbooks and interest in herbalism increased rapidly. The first major English work on botanical medicine was the *Rosa Medicinae* written by a monk, John of Gaddesden, between 1314 and 1317. This was also the age of exploration and the discovery of central America in 1492, led by Christopher Columbus, resulted in an increase in the variety and number of imported herbs and spices available throughout Europe.

More and more authoritative and comprehensive herbals were produced. In 1551, William Turner, who was the first person to study plants scientifically, produced the *New Herball*, John Gerard's extremely popular *Herball* was published in 1597. This well-known Elizabethan herbalist had a garden in London where he grew plants he had collected from all over the world.

In the sixteenth century, the Doctrine of Signatures, promoted by a German physician called Paracelsus, proved to be very influential. The basis of his theory was that the appearance of a plant gave an indication of the ailments it would cure. For example, the root of the saffron, considered to look like a deformed gouty foot, was believed to be an effective cure for gout. There was a degree of truth in this theory in that the root is a rich source of a painkiller useful in the treatment of pain that accompanies conditions such as gout. However, the Doctrine of Signatures theory didn't prove quite so satisfactory with all herbs.

The Complete Herbal, written by Nicholas Culpeper in 1649, was an immediate success. It has been reprinted many times and is still in print today. Culpeper, an apothecary, was the first herbalist to write in English for ordinary people rather than in Latin which was used by physicians. His herbal allowed patients to go out and collect their herbs from the countryside and prepare their own remedies or obtain Culpeper's own plant medicines at very low cost instead of paying vastly inflated apothecary bills. Today, Culpeper gives its name to a company founded by Mrs C.F. Leyel (who also established the Society of Herbalists) in 1927, which sells a range of natural herbal products in a number of outlets throughout the country.

Although herbs were still the main source of medicine, Paracelsus had already developed the idea of using chemical compounds in medicine by introducing elements, such as iron and mercury, into medical practice. Gradually, during the seventeenth and eighteenth centuries, the skills of herbalists were replaced by medical techniques that owed more to the scientific laboratory than to traditional practices.

In 1785, English physician William Withering discovered that foxglove leaves had great success in treating dropsy and heart failure. When analysed by scientists the active ingredients of digoxin and digitoxin contained within the plant were identified as providing the effective remedy. These two active constituents were then isolated, extracted, and then reproduced synthetically and are still used in treating heart conditions today.

This process was subsequently applied to other valuable properties discovered in plants, which were found to have medicinal and therapeutic benefits, and are the basis of many of today's modern medicines. Other plant-derived drugs of today include morphine from the opium poppy and the anti-malarial quinine, which originally came from the Peruvian fever tree, cinchona.

In the last quarter of the twentieth century there can be no doubt about the dominance of chemical medicine with the breakthrough of such 'wonder drugs' as antibiotics. However, concern grows about the numerous side effects that often accompany such modern orthodox drugs – a recent study revealed that two out of five people receiving clinical drugs suffer side effects, which in many cases are much more serious than the condition being treated – and, in some cases, the failure of such orthodox drugs to treat certain degenerative and stress-related illnesses. These concerns combined with today's greater awareness of environmental issues, means interest in herbal medicine is increasing throughout the Western world.

As with medicine, there is also an increasing demand for more natural cosmetics. Beauty houses the world over are being compelled by public demand to use more natural ingredients – which are just as effective as synthetic substitutes but don't carry the potential risk of side effects – in their products and fewer of those manufactured by the chemicals industry. This is clearly demonstrated by the growth of environmentally aware companies such as Body Shop, Cosmetics To Go and Montagne Jeunesse, who are all committed to using natural, plant-based ingredients in their range of beauty products.

Research is continually being carried out to identify and learn more about the active constituents contained within plants that give them their healing and therapeutic proper-ties so beneficial to the body. A chance discovery in the 1950s revealed that the Madagascan periwinkle, a rain-forest plant, had beneficial effects in the treatment of leukaemia through its effect on the body's white blood cells. However, few wild specimens of the plant remain in its native Madagascar. Another cancer drug obtained from a plant was etoposide, extracted from the American Mayapple. Other proven success stories include the use of the herb feverfew in the treatment of migraine and evening primrose which has shown to have considerable success in the treatment of eczema and premenstrual tension. This particular plant is also being investigated in relation to its healing potential in a wide range of other conditions from multiple sclerosis to schizophrenia.

Other plants currently under investigation include the Australian Moreton Bay Chestnut for its effects on the immune system; echinacea and myrrh in relation to their possible role in the treatment of AIDS; hawthorn in the treatment of angina, heart failure, hypertension and coronary thrombosis; and the anti-cancer activity of garlic, which is also being studied for its effects in lowering blood pressure and cholesterol levels.

The medical herbalists, or phytotherapists, of today are not only experts in the traditional use of herbal medicine but also in its biochemistry and pharmacology, and they are able to use their training in conventional medical science within the context of a holistic approach to healing.

In the cosmetics industry also, plants and their beneficial therapeutic properties are being closely examined. Body Shop founder Anita Roddick travels the world researching the natural raw materials used by various native communities for personal health and bodycare. In Tahiti, for example, she was introduced to the custom of using mud to cleanse the hair and cocoa butter to protect the skin. Her company, along with other environmentally conscious organisations working towards protecting and conserving natural resources, follow a policy of trade not aid by offering products to local communities in exchange for the natural, raw ingredients found in their area and also by putting a proportion of profits back to help support the communities and their natural environments.

The process of examining and researching plants for their medicinal and therapeutic uses continues throughout the world. In 1992, the European Scientific Cooperative for Phytotherapy (ESCOP), which includes the British Herbal Medicine Association and other comparable organisations from Belgium, France, Germany, the Netherlands and Switzerland, began a major European research project to study the effectiveness of herbal medicines and to provide scientific validation. Their task is awesome. It is estimated that only 10 per cent of higher plants have so far been studied scientifically. In Brazil, for example, there are considered to be some 55,000 species of higher plant and nothing is known about 99 per cent of them. The problem is that time is running out as more and more plant species are in danger of becoming extinct, especially in the tropical rain forests which are being tragically decimated. Dr Linda Fellows, head of the biochemistry section at the Royal Botanic Gardens, Kew, says, 'With the current rate of destruction it is estimated about one-fifth of rain forest plant species would probably be lost within the next 50 years if something is not done.'

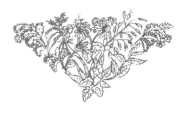

2

Preparing herbs

There are a number of different ways to prepare herbs for use in health and beauty herbal remedies. For most of the recipes in this book you can use either fresh herbs, depending on availability, or dried herbs. Prepare your remedies daily rather than make up large quantities to store. Depending on the active constituents they contain, dried green herbs may lose their potency quicker than roots, seeds and bark.

Harvesting and drying

Growing and collecting your own herbs will not only give you a decorative array of aromatic plants, but it will also ensure the quality of your plants. Most herbs are easy to grow and many will flourish in pots on a balcony or patio, or even indoors.

The quality of the herb is most important. When using fresh plants for herbal remedies, pick perfect leaves, clean and unblemished, at their prime time which is when most of their active constituents are present. In general, leaves reach their peak just before their flowers open; flowers reach their peak just as they open; fruit as it becomes ripe but before it becomes too soft to dry effectively; roots in the autumn when the aerial parts of the plant have died down (with the exception of dandelion root which should be gathered in the spring) and bark after the spring when the sap is falling. When collecting bark, never remove all the bark, or an entire band from a tree, or it will kill the tree, and always dust or wipe bark thoroughly to remove any moss or insects before drying.

There are strict laws regarding the picking of wild plants. Some may be on the endangered species list, which means to pick them is strictly prohibited, and even those not in danger of becoming extinct cannot be collected without first asking the landowner's permission.

Ideally, collect your herbs on a dry sunny morning, once the dew has dried as any dampness will cause them to deteriorate quickly. Never pick herbs that grow within 40–50 feet of a road as they will be contaminated by exhaust fumes. Plants growing near cultivated fields that have been sprayed should also be avoided. An accurate identification of the herbs is also vital as some plants are poisonous at all times and others can be harmful if the recommended guidelines are not followed. If in doubt, always seek expert advice. Dried herbs can easily be bought from health food shops or through specialist suppliers, a selection of which can be found towards the end of the book.

If drying your own fresh herbs, it's important that the valuable volatile oils, that contain the plant's medicinal and therapeutic properties, are not lost. Large leaves can be picked individually for drying whilst smaller leaves are best left on the stem. Carefully wipe off any soil or grit and avoid rinsing unless absolutely necessary. Tie the aerial parts of the plant or large leaves in small bunches and hang upside down to dry, or spread out flatly in one single layer on a paper-lined tray in a warm, well-ventilated place, such as an airing cupboard with the door open. Avoid using a garage as the herbs may become contaminated by petrol fumes. When drying roots, wash thoroughly and chop into small pieces before spreading out to dry. Turn the herbs frequently over the next few days, especially fleshy fruit (discard fruit with any signs of mould), to ensure even drying and, when dry, break them up into small pieces.

Generally, herbs should be completely dry within six days. Leaves should be brittle and break easily; stems and stalks should break and not bend; flower petals should be dry without crumbling; and bark and roots should be dry enough to snap into manageable pieces or, if they are thick they can be broken up with a small hammer. Dried herbs should look, taste and smell like the fresh plant but be about one-eighth of the weight.

When dry, store the herbs in sterilised, dry dark glass or pottery airtight containers away from direct sunlight. Never store in plastic bags or containers as this will encourage condensation. Be sure to label and date all your prepared herbs carefully. Leaves and flowers, when dried, will keep for about 12–18 months, roots and bark for about two years.

Getting herbs ready for action

The methods of preparing herbs for use in the herbal remedies that follow all use standard quantities of herb. Throughout the book all quantities and doses are the recommended standard for adults unless otherwise specified. For medicinal herbal remedies for children and the elderly, doses should be reduced depending on age, see Chapter 4, Herbs for health, on page 55. Where a remedy uses a combination of herbs, the total amount of herbs used should not exceed the standard quantity.

Useful measuring equivalents

Liquid	*Solids*
1 ml = 20 drops	10 g = 1 tsp
5 ml = 1 tsp	30 g = 1 (heaped) tblsp
20 ml = 1 tblsp	
75 ml = ½ cup	
150 ml = 1 cup	

Store preparations in sterilised bottles or jars with plastic screwtops (not metal) and keep in the fridge or a cool place, unless specified. Small stoppered jars using corks or plastic corks are an alternative.

Infusion

This method is best when using the soft, aerial parts of the plant like the leaves or flowers. Making an infusion is just like making tea. Warm a pot or cup and add the required amount of fresh or dried herb. For a standard infusion use:

- 90 g (3 tblsp) fresh or 30 g (1 tblsp) dried finely chopped herb to 500 ml of water.

or when making an individual cup, use:

- 30 g (1 tblsp) fresh or 10 g (1 tsp) finely chopped herb to 150 ml (1 cup) of water.

Pour over water just off the boil – boiling water disperses valuable volatile oils in the steam – and cover. Leave to infuse for 10–15 minutes, then strain through either a fine sieve, muslin or a jelly bag into an airtight container. Use within two or three days. When used as a medicinal remedy, a herbal infusion can be taken hot or cold. When taken internally, hot infusions are naturally warming and often promote perspiration.

Decoction

This method is recommended when using the hard, woody parts of a herb, such as the root, bark, stem or seed. These all have tough cell walls that require prolonged heat to break them down so that their active components can be released.

Chop or break up the fresh or dried herb into manageable pieces. For a standard decoction use:

*   90g (3 tblsp) fresh or 30g (1 tblsp) dried herb to 750ml water, reduced to around 500ml after heating.

Measure the required amount of herb into an enamel or stainless steel pan. (Do not use an aluminium or non-stick pan, as contact with these surfaces may destroy some of the active constituents of the herb.) Cover with the cold water, bring to the boil and simmer for between 30 minutes to one hour, until the liquid has been reduced by one third. Strain and when cool pour into sterilised bottles or jars. Decoctions will keep for two days if stored in the fridge, but should be drunk hot when used as a medicinal remedy.

Some herbs used in infusions or decoctions may taste bitter. To combat this either sweeten with a little honey or combine with another more pleasant tasting herb in the infusion or decoction, making sure that the plants are compatible with each other and don't interact. Aromatic herbs such as peppermint, lemon balm, lavender, catnip and fennel will disguise the taste of less palatable herbs.

Note
With the herbs marshmallow and valerian, the infusion should be made with cold water, as warm water may extract some inactive constituents in the plant and therefore alter its content.

Tincture

These mixtures are alcoholic extracts of herb, and the amount used is much smaller than with infusions or decoctions. As well as extracting the plant's active ingredients, the alcohol acts as a preservative. Therefore tinctures have a much longer shelf life and will keep for up to two years. To make a standard tincture use:

- 240g fresh or 120g dried finely chopped herb to 500ml of alcohol with a strength of between 25 per cent and 45 per cent, such as gin or vodka.

Place the herb into a large, sterilised screwtop jar and cover with the alcohol. Store in a warm place out of direct sunlight for two weeks, shaking well once a day. Then strain through fine muslin or a jelly bag, squeezing out as much liquid as you can. Then store in sterilised dark glass bottles. If taken internally the recommended dosage of tincture should always be diluted in a little water.

Tinctures can also be added to infusions, compresses or the bath.

Compress

A method to use when applying a herbal remedy externally to the skin. For a hot compress, soak a piece of clean cotton cloth in a hot standard infusion or decoction or 5–20ml (1–4 tsp) of tincture. Squeeze out the excess liquid and apply to the affected area. Cover with a folded towel to keep in the heat. Replace when cooled. Prepare a cold compress in the same way but allow to cool before applying.

Poultice

This is similar to a compress, except that the actual herb is used rather than a liquid extraction. Mash or crush sufficient plant parts to cover the affected area. If you are using dried herb, mix to a thick paste with a little water or cider vinegar. Then heat the pulp or paste in a pan over boiling water or mix with a small amount of boiling water. Apply a little oil to the skin beforehand to prevent the herb sticking, and then either apply the pulp directly to the skin, as hot as it can be tolerated, holding it in place with a gauze bandage, or put the pulp between two layers of muslin cloth and then apply it to the affected area. Change when it cools. A hot water bottle placed over the poultice on the affected area will help keep the heat in longer.

Ointment

Melt 250g of vegetable fat or cocoa butter over a pan of boiling water or in a double saucepan. Stir in 30g (1 tblsp) of dried herb and heat gently for about two hours or until the herb is crisp, checking from time to time that the water doesn't run dry. Pour the mixture through muslin or a jelly bag into a jug and, while warm, quickly pour the strained mixture into sterilised glass storage jars and leave to set. A drop of tincture of myrrh added to the blended mixture before it cools will help prolong its shelf life. If kept in a fridge, it should keep for a couple of months.

Infused herbal oil

Some active plant ingredients can be extracted in oil for external use. An infused oil can be made with the fresh or dried parts of the herb and will keep for up to a year, depending on the plant used. Store in a dark, cool place. Herbal infused oils can be made two ways.

The cold technique

Pack a large screwtop, sterilised glass jar with the finely chopped, fresh or dried herb of your choice. Cover with oil (use sunflower, olive or almond oil – the latter is best if it is to be used for cosmetic purposes), seal and put in a warm place. Leave for two weeks, shaking the jar well each day. The oil will take up the components of the herbs. Strain the mixture through muslin or a jelly bag. Pour into sterilised, airtight bottles, store and label.

The hot technique

Put 500 ml sunflower oil and 750 g fresh or 250 g dried herb in a bowl over a pan of hot water and heat gently for three hours. Strain the mixture through muslin or a jelly bag and pour into sterilised, airtight storage bottles and label.

Syrup

A syrup makes the more unpleasant tasting herbs more palatable. Warm 200 ml of your selected strained standard infusion or decoction over a gentle heat with 200 g of sugar until the sugar is dissolved and the mixture turns syrupy. Allow the mixture to cool and pour into a dark glass sterilised bottle. Seal with a cork stopper (screwtop bottles can explode if the syrup ferments) and store in a dark, cool place.

Inhalation

Half fill a bowl with a standard hot infusion or decoction, or put 30–60g (1–2 tblsp) of dried herb in the bowl and cover with boiling water. Lean over the bowl and cover your head and the bowl with a towel to trap in the steam. Breathe slowly and deeply to reap the benefit of the herbal vapour for 5–10 minutes. Repeat twice a day.

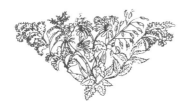

The beauty of herbs

3

Since ancient times, plants have been used to beautify and enhance. Recipes for herbal cosmetic preparations have been handed down from generation to generation – from the early Egyptians, who would anoint their dead both to preserve the body and make it beautiful for the next world, to the Romans who developed a wide range of recipes for bleaching, tinting and greasing hair, for avoiding wrinkles and promoting a fine complexion and for masking body odour.

Today, the man-made cosmetics business is a multi-million pound industry. Products don't come cheap and the increased use of chemical preservatives, artificial colourings and synthetic perfumes, which often provoke allergic reactions in sensitive skins, has prompted a growing number of people to look for more natural products to use on their body, face and hair.

Making your own cosmetics using the therapeutic properties of herbs can be interesting and fun. Herbal beauty products are simple to prepare and are effective without being terribly expensive. Herbs are easy to obtain or even grow yourself. And by making your own products you can be sure they are completely safe and natural. You select each ingredient and have control over its freshness and purity. Quite apart from anything else, the glorious fragrance of the herbs will, in itself, have such a beneficial soothing or stimulating effect, you can't help but feel more beautiful!

Obviously healthy, beautiful-looking skin and hair cannot be obtained by using cosmetic preparations alone, whatever their ingredients. It is also important to have a well-balanced diet, get sufficient sleep, do plenty of exercise and make time for relaxation in order to ensure that the herbal preparations you use are fully effective.

It is also important to remember that, without the chemical preservatives of proprietary cosmetics, home-made herbal products do not have as long a shelf life. As a general rule, make up each preparation on the day you want to use it where possible, rather than making a large quantity and storing it. Make sure all storage bottles and jars are clean and thoroughly sterilised in boiling water before use. Always keep home-made cosmetics in the fridge away from food, or, where specified, store in a dark, cool place such as a cupboard. Don't forget to label each jar or bottle with details of the contents and date.

All remedies in this chapter and throughout the book use standard quantities of herb, as given in Chapter 2, Preparing herbs (see p. 11), unless otherwise stated. When using a combination of herbs, the total amount should not exceed the standard recommended quantity.

Before making any herbal preparation, always look up the particular herb(s) you want to use in Chapter 5, The A–Z of herbs (see pages 97–140) for a complete plant profile and take note of any cautions. Then refer to Chapter 2, Preparing herbs (see pages 11–19) for how to prepare your chosen herb for use in the remedy, if appropriate.

Note

Whenever a recipe recommends using nettle for use on the hair or body, if using the fresh plant, handle with extreme care. Wear gloves to avoid being stung and boil the plant to eliminate the sting. It is also important always to carry out a small skin test with all the herbal cosmetic preparations before use, to make sure that there is no allergic reaction. Apply a small amount of your chosen remedy to the skin. If there is no allergic reaction after 12 hours, go ahead and use the preparation.

FACE

Herbal skin savers

Recommended herbs

Normal skin	Dry/sensitive skin	Oily skin	Mature/ sallow skin
Fennel	Elderflower	Chamomile	Dandelion
Fumitory	Marigold	Chickweed	Elderflower
Horsetail	Marshmallow	Sage	Lavender
Lady's mantle		Yarrow	
Lime flowers			
Nettle			
Peppermint			
St John's wort			

Handy herbal beauty basics

Cleansers

Apply morning and night. Put a little of the lotion or milk into the palm of one hand, rub hands together and massage gently into the face. Or with a cream, simply put a couple of small blobs onto the face and massage in. Tissue off using gentle, upward movements.

Herbal cleansing lotion

Simmer one handful of fresh or 10g (1 tsp) of dried chosen herb, finely chopped in 250ml water for 10–15 minutes. Strain and cool. Use daily. Store in fridge and use within two to three days.

Herbal cleansing milk

Put 30g (1 tblsp) of fresh or 10g (1 tsp) of dried chosen herb(s), finely chopped, in 150ml (1 cup) of boiling water and leave to steep for 10 minutes. Strain. Take 10g (1 tsp) of cornflour and mix to a smooth paste with a small amount of the infusion. Stir in 8ml (1½ tsp) of fresh milk and 5ml (1 tsp) sunflower oil and then gradually mix in the rest of the infusion. Warm to boiling point. Remove from heat and leave to cool. Apply daily. Keep in fridge and use within two to three days.

Herbal toner

Apply morning and night on a pad of cotton wool with gentle, upward movements. This will help tighten the pores after cleansing and also help stimulate the circulation.

Pour 150ml (1 cup) of boiling water over 30g (1 tblsp) of fresh or 10g (1 tsp) of dried chopped herb(s) and leave to infuse for 20 minutes. Strain and cool. Use daily after cleansing. Keep in the fridge and use within two to three days.

Herbal moisturiser

Apply night and morning. Place a very small amount in the palm of one hand, rub hands together and then massage the moisturiser onto the face, being careful not to pull or drag the skin. You will need:

- 2–3 very soft, fresh apricots, chopped (if using dried, soften first in cold water for one hour, then strain and chop before using)
- 75ml (½ cup) and 40ml (2 tblsp) glycerine
- a pinch of fresh or dried St John's wort, finely chopped or ground
- a pinch of fresh or dried marigold flowers, crumbled
- 15g (½ tblsp) cornflour
- 20ml (1 tblsp) light sunflower oil

- 120ml (6 tblsp) water (for normal and dry/sensitive skins substitute the water for orange flower water. For oily skins substitute the water for rose water.)

Mash the apricots and blend with the 75ml (½ cup) glycerine, or pop both into a blender and liquidise for a couple of minutes. Add the herbs. Stir well and then push through a sieve. Blend the cornflour with the sunflower oil into a smooth paste. Gradually stir in the 40ml (2 tblsp) glycerine and the water. Blend with the apricot mixture and then warm to boiling point, stirring occasionally, until smooth and thickened. Cool. Keep in the fridge and use within four days.

Deep cleansing face pack

A weekly, deep cleansing face pack or mask will remove all traces of stale make-up and help keep the complexion radiant and clear. Apply to slightly damp skin, ideally after steaming. You will need:

- 20ml (1 tblsp) natural yogurt
- 20ml (1 tblsp) honey
- 30g (1 tblsp) fresh or 10g (1 tsp) dried herb
- 75ml (½ cup) boiling water
- medium oatmeal, wheatgerm or Fuller's Earth

Blend yogurt with honey. Steep your chosen herb in the boiling water and leave for half an hour. Do not strain. Add 20ml (1 tblsp) of the infusion to the yogurt and honey. Blend well and then thicken to a stiff paste by stirring in either a little oatmeal, wheatgerm or Fuller's Earth. Gently apply to the face and neck, carefully avoiding the delicate area around the eyes. Leave on for 15 minutes before rinsing off with warm water and moisturising. Keep in the fridge and use within three days.

Herbal deep cleansing mask

For normal skins

Liquidise or mash a slice of soft, fresh pineapple with 113 ml (¾ cup) of glycerine. Add 5 g (½ tsp) of each of the following fresh or dried herbs: lady's mantle, lime flowers, nettle (must be dried), peppermint. Mix to a paste with kaolin – use approximately one part of the fruit mixture to five parts of kaolin. Spread gently over the face and neck, carefully avoiding the eye area. Leave on for about 15 minutes and remove with lukewarm water. Keep in the fridge and use within three days. Enough for two to three applications.

For dry/sensitive skins

Liquidise or mash a slice of soft, fresh pineapple with 38 ml (¼ cup) of glycerine. Add 5 g (½ tsp) of fresh or dried marshmallow. If using marshmallow root, boil it for 5–10 minutes first and crush to extract a mucilage (a gel-like substance) and add this. Mix to a paste with kaolin and apply and store as above.

For oily skins

Follow instructions for normal skin, replacing the pineapple with half a peeled lemon. The recommended herbs to use are 10 g (1 tsp) each of fresh or dried sage and yarrow.

Herbal exfoliator

This is basically a way of polishing the skin. An exfoliator works by gently rubbing away the dead cells, which accumulate on the surface of the skin, and by helping to stimulate the production of new cells. This improves the texture of the skin, leaving it smooth and glowing. Simply mix a little medium oatmeal with a little of your chosen standard herbal infusion into a paste. Then rub onto your face using small, circular movements. This should be done once a week before cleansing. It is not recommended for highly sensitive skin as it can prove too harsh and cause irritation.

Herbal skin treats

Herbal facial steam

After cleansing, a facial steam opens the pores and helps get rid of ingrained impurities. It also leaves the facial muscles relaxed and makes your skin more receptive for further treatments, such as a face pack. Do not have a facial steam if you have a tendency to broken veins and always protect the delicate area around the eyes with a thin layer of moisturiser.

Recommended herbs

Deep cleansing	Dry/sensitive skin	Oily skin
Chamomile	Lady's mantle	Herb Robert
Fennel	Marshmallow	Horsetail
Lime flowers	Parsley	Sage
Nettle		Yarrow
Rosemary		

Mature/sallow skin	Blackheads/problem skin
Dandelion	Burdock
Elderflower	Chamomile
Lavender	Elecampane
	Lemon balm
	Lime flowers
	Valerian

Place 30g (1 tblsp) fresh or 10g (1 tsp) dried of your chosen herb(s), (you can use a combination of the recommended herbs for your skin type) in a large bowl or sink and then pour on boiling water until half full. Hold your face over the bowl and cover your head and the bowl or sink with a towel to trap in the steam. Hold for about five minutes and then pat skin dry with a towel. For best results always gently steam your face before applying a face pack. If you aren't applying a face pack, simply moisturise.

Rosemary skin booster
A stimulating tonic with a wonderful aroma to really awaken tired skin, leaving it feeling tingly and fresh. Use straight from the fridge first thing in the morning to kickstart the circulation into action. You will need:

- 90g (3 tblsp) fresh or 30g (1 tblsp) dried rosemary, finely chopped
- 500ml hot water
- 20ml (4 tsp) of a 37.5 per cent alcohol such as gin or vodka

Put the finely chopped rosemary into the hot water, cover and simmer for 10 minutes. Remove from heat and leave to steep for one hour. Strain, and when cool add the gin or vodka to the infusion. Bottle, shake well and store in the fridge, it will keep for three to four days. Apply on cotton wool pads after cleansing.

Sage and marigold astringent
A must for oily and problem skin – this herby astringent will not only help put a stop to troublesome spots, but by acting as a great skin pick-me-up it will also tone and refine the complexion. You will need:

- a pinch each of fresh or dried sage and marigold flowers
- 75 ml (½ cup) boiling water
- distilled witch hazel, in equal parts to the sage and marigold infusion

Add the herbs to the boiling water. Steep for 30 minutes. Strain and cool before adding the distilled witch hazel. Apply on cotton wool pads after cleansing. Store in the fridge and use within four days.

Elderflower and honey facial scrub

Revitalise dull-looking skin with a twice weekly facial scrub. You will need:

- 30g (1 tblsp) fresh or 10g (1 tsp) dried elderflowers, finely chopped
- 75 ml (½ cup) boiling water
- 10 ml (½ tblsp) clear honey
- 8 ml (1½ tsp) milk
- 10g (1 tsp) ground almonds
- 38 ml (¼ cup) fine oatmeal
- 5 ml (1 tsp) cider vinegar

Make an infusion by steeping the elderflowers in the boiling water. Do not strain, just leave for half an hour. Mix together clear honey, milk, ground almonds, ground oatmeal and cider vinegar until well blended. Stir in 20 ml (1 tblsp) of the elderflower infusion. Store in a sealed plastic container in the fridge. It should keep for four to five days. To use, place a small amount in the palm of the hand, moisten with a little water and apply to cleansed skin in small circular movements around the neck and face, avoiding the delicate eye area. Wash off with tepid water, pat skin dry and apply moisturiser.

Peppermint and marigold compress for enlarged pores

Peppermint is a mild astringent and antiseptic and, combined with the antibacterial and antiseptic properties of marigold, makes an effective skin tonic that will help tighten enlarged pores. You will need:

- 10g (1 tsp) each of fresh or dried marigold flowers and peppermint
- 75ml (½ cup) boiling water

Put marigold and peppermint in boiling water. Leave to infuse for 20 minutes. Strain and cool slightly. While still warm, soak cotton wool pads in the liquid, squeeze out excess liquid and apply to clean skin, being careful not to pull or drag the skin. Keep in the fridge for two to three days.

Plantain problem skin lotion

Plantain is a cleansing herb and will help keep the skin healthy and blemish-free. You will need:

- 10g (1 tsp) dried plantain (plantago major) leaves
- 150ml (1 cup) boiling water

Put plantain leaves in a bowl and add boiling water. Leave to infuse for one hour. Strain and apply the lotion with cotton wool daily. Store in the fridge and use within three days.

Lime flowers and avocado rich moisture cream

Nurture the skin as you sleep with this rich, moisturising night cream using lime flowers known for their wonderful aroma and skin softening properties. You will need:

- 30g (1 tblsp) fresh or 10g (1 tsp) dried lime flowers

- 150ml (1 cup) boiling water
- ¼ ripe, soft avocado
- 20ml (1 tblsp) natural yogurt
- 20ml (1 tblsp) single cream

Make an infusion of lime flowers by adding the flowers to the boiling water. Leave to infuse for one hour until cool. Do not strain. Mash the ripe avocado and mix with natural yogurt, single cream and 40ml (2 tblsp) of the lime flowers infusion. Pour the mixture into a container, seal tightly and keep in the fridge for two to three days. Massage a very small amount into the face and neck last thing at night until fully absorbed and leave it on while you sleep for maximum hydration. Rinse your face first thing in the morning before cleansing.

Lavender anti-blemish night cream
Let the antiseptic and slightly cooling properties of lavender get to work while you sleep on treating skin prone to blemishes, spots and pimples. You will need:

- 150ml (1 cup) boiling water
- 30g (1 tblsp) fresh or 10g (1 tsp) dried lavender flowers
- 30g (1 tblsp) soya flour
- 160ml (8 tblsp) safflower oil
- juice of ¼ lemon
- 45g (1½ tblsp) parsley, finely chopped
- 5g (½ tsp) salt
- 5g (½ tsp) fresh chamomile flowers

First of all make up a lavender infusion by pouring the boiling water over the lavender. Leave to infuse for two hours, then strain. Bottle the water and keep in the fridge for future use. Mix the soya flour with 30ml (1½ tblsp) lavender water to a smooth paste and place in a small bowl over a saucepan of hot water. Beat in the safflower oil and whisk until it thickens. Remove from heat and add the lemon juice, parsley, salt and fresh chamomile flowers. Blend the mixture for a few minutes until creamy. Leave to cool, then transfer into a small airtight container. Store in the fridge and use within three to four days. Apply a very small amount last thing at night, after applying your herbal cleanser and astringent. Blot with tissue to remove excess.

Cowslip anti-wrinkle lotion
You will need:

- 75 ml (½ cup) boiling water
- 30 g (1 tblsp) fresh or 10 g (1 tsp) dried cowslip flowers

Pour boiling water onto the cowslip flowers. Leave to infuse for five minutes. Strain and cool. Soak cotton wool pads or balls in the cool infusion, shake off any excess liquid and apply gently to the lines and wrinkles as a smoothing compress. Leave for five minutes then repeat. Bottle and store in the fridge for up to two to three days.

Elderflower toner for thread veins
You will need:

- 150 ml (1 cup) boiling water
- 30 g (1 tblsp) fresh or 10 g (1 tsp) dried elderflowers

Pour the water over the flowers and leave to infuse for one to two hours. Strain and store in the fridge for two to three days. Use the lotion night and morning to help dilated veins.

Dandelion freckle oil
This dandelion oil will help naturally bleach and fade away

stubborn freckles, brown age spots and small, light moles. You will need:

- 4 medium-sized dandelion leaves
- 100ml (5 tblsp) castor oil

Wash and chop the dandelion leaves and place them in a small pan with the castor oil. Heat gently and simmer for 10 minutes. Remove from the heat. Cover and leave to infuse for three hours. Strain, bottle and label. Gently apply a very small amount of the oil to the skin daily. If kept in a fridge, this infused oil should keep for a month.

EYES

Plenty of sleep together with a well-balanced diet are vital if you want to have beautiful, sparkling eyes. However, herbs can also be useful for helping to ease eyes that are tired or have become bloodshot, sore or inflamed. A number of herbs are known for their soothing and anti-inflammatory action, while others will certainly help keep eyes clear, bright and sparkling.

Recommended herbs

Soothes tired, sore and inflamed eyes	Reduces puffiness and adds sparkle	Minimises dark circles
Chamomile	Elderflower	Peppermint
Eyebright	Eyebright	
Horsetail	Fennel seed	
Marigold		

Note
For all eye solutions, always simmer herbs in boiling water for 10–15 minutes to make sure any bacteria is destroyed and strain the solution three times through fine muslin cloth or a jelly bag. This is to make sure no small particles get through which may cause irritation to the eyes. Always use a fresh cotton wool pad or cucumber slice for each eye and each application.

Herbal eye bath

Add 60g (2 tblsp) fresh or 20g (2 tsp) dried herb(s) to 300ml (2 cups) of water and bring to the boil, then simmer gently for 10–15 minutes and then remove from heat. Leave for 30 minutes and then strain thoroughly. Either use directly as an eye bath, or soak cotton wool pads or thick slices of cucumber in the liquid, shake off excess liquid and apply to the eyes as a compress. Lie down and relax for 10 minutes in a darkened room. Do not keep the infusion – throw away and make fresh for each application.

Herbal eye treats

Eyebright eye gel

Add 30g (1 tblsp) fresh or 10g (1 tsp) dried eyebright leaves to 250ml of cold water and bring to the boil. Simmer for 10–15 minutes. Cover and leave to steep for about five minutes before straining. Use this decoction to make up half a sachet of gelatine (following the instructions on the packet) and leave to set to produce a soothing and cooling eye gel. Store in the fridge and use within three days.

Rosemary puffy eyes lotion

Make up a standard decoction of rosemary using 30g (1 tblsp) fresh or 10g (1 tsp) dried herb to 150ml (1 cup) of boiling water, and simmer gently for 10 minutes. Leave to stand for 30 minutes and then strain thoroughly. Apply cool on cotton wool pads, pressing lightly onto the delicate puffy areas. Use after cleansing the face in the morning. Store in the fridge and use within two to three days.

MOUTH

The cleansing, antiseptic and refreshing properties of many herbs make them ideal when it comes to looking after your teeth and gums.

Herbal breath fresheners

To freshen the breath and neutralise strong odours, chew – but don't swallow – either fresh, clean parsley, aniseed or peppermint leaves. Fresh, clean sage leaves rubbed over the teeth and gums will leave them feeling clean and polished.

Herbal treats for the mouth

Witch hazel gargle

A quick and easy mouthwash to freshen up the mouth. Once bottled add a few sprigs of fresh peppermint or lemon or orange peel. You will need:

- 60ml (3 tblsp) distilled witch hazel
- 300ml (2 cups) still mineral water

Mix the ingredients together and store in a screwtop bottle. Rinse the mouth, without swallowing. Use within one week, as required.

Peppermint and raspberry mouthwash

You will need:

- 5 sprigs fresh peppermint leaves (use the tender ends of stems with 5–6 leaves on each) finely chopped
- 5 fresh raspberries, mashed to a pulp
- 75ml (½ cup) glycerine
- still mineral water

Add the peppermint leaves and raspberries to the glycerine. Mix well (or liquidise) and strain through a muslin cloth or a jelly bag. Mix equal parts of this mixture with equal parts of still mineral water and use to rinse the mouth, without swallowing. Use within one to two days.

Peppermint toothpaste

The mixture cleans the teeth and freshens the mouth. Use with a damp toothbrush. You will need:

- 3 sprigs of fresh peppermint leaves (use the tender ends of stems with 5–6 leaves on each) finely chopped
- 38 ml (¼ cup) of boiling water
- 3 ml (½ tsp) sunflower oil
- 3 g (¼ tsp) cornflour
- 10 ml (½ tblsp) glycerine

Steep the fresh peppermint leaves in the boiling water in a thermos flask for 30 minutes. Strain. Mix the sunflower oil and cornflour into a smooth paste and add 20 ml (1 tblsp) of the strained peppermint infusion and 10 ml (½ tblsp) glycerine. Bring to the boil. Cool and stir occasionally. Use this paste within one day.

Apricot, banana and sage lip balm

A fruity lip balm to keep your lips super smooth. Use as often as possible and before applying lipstick to stop it from 'bleeding'. You will need:

- ½ soft banana
- 2 fresh, chopped apricots (you can use dried, but soften in water for one hour and strain before using)
- 75 ml (½ cup) of almond oil
- 10 g (1 tsp) dried sage
- vegetable fat, softened

Mash the banana and apricots and mix well with the almond oil and dried sage – or liquidise everything in a blender. Stir thoroughly and push through a fine sieve. Melt vegetable fat – use an amount equal to that of the filtered fruit and almond oil mixture – in a heavy-bottomed saucepan over a gentle heat. When melted, remove from the heat and gradually stir in the oil mixture. Blend thoroughly, pour into a small jar and leave to set. Store in fridge and use within two weeks.

HAIR

The condition of your hair is often an indication of the state of your overall well-being. A poor diet, lack of sleep, too much stress, and hormonal changes, can all take their toll and cause problems for your hair. So it's vital to maintain a healthy lifestyle in order to keep your locks looking healthy too.

However, other factors such as over-exposure to the sun, chemical treatments and dyes, central heating and environmental pollution can also damage hair, leaving it looking dull and out of condition. So, whatever type of hair you have, it needs constant care and attention to keep it in peak condition.

The majority of proprietary shampoos and haircare products sold over the counter today have a synthetic base which, if used on a regular basis, can often be too harsh on the hair. They can strip it of its natural acidity, leaving it dull-looking and lifeless. However, your own totally natural, home-made herbal preparations, with their gentle cleansing action, won't upset the hair's pH balance and, in conjunction with a healthy diet and lifestyle can have incredible results, giving the hair vital shine, body and bounce.

Handy herbal basics for hair

Recommended herbs for shampoo/conditioners

Normal	Dry/sensitive	Oily
Catnip	Burdock	Elderflower
Fennel	Chamomile	Lavender
Horsetail	Lime flowers	Marigold
Nettle	Marshmallow	Peppermint
	Parsley	Rosemary
	Sage	Witch hazel
		Yarrow

Anti-dandruff	For shine and lustre	Improved growth
Burdock	Cleavers	Catnip
Cleavers	Horsetail	Nettle
Elderflower	Lime flowers	Thyme
Horsetail	Marigold	
Lavender	Nettle	
Marigold	Parsley	
Peppermint	Rosemary	
Rosemary	Sage	
Sage		
Witch hazel		
Yarrow		

Herbal shampoo

Pour one application of a mild baby shampoo into a cup and add 40ml (2 tblsp) of a standard infusion or decoction of your chosen herb. Mix well. After rinsing your hair with warm water, apply a small amount of shampoo to your palm and gently massage it through the hair and into the scalp. Rinse with warm water. Repeat and give hair a final rinse in cool water to remove any last traces of shampoo and to tone the scalp.

Herbal conditioner

Beat one egg and stir in 3 ml (½ tsp) honey. Steep 5 g (½ tsp) of your chosen finely chopped herb, fresh or dried, in 75 ml (½ cup) of boiling water. Leave to infuse for 10 minutes, then strain and cool. Add the infusion to the egg mixture and blend in. Massage through the hair – paying particular attention to the ends – and onto the scalp after washing. Leave for five minutes and then rinse off thoroughly with warm water.

Herbal tonic finishing rinse

A good hair tonic will help give hair body, keep it glossy and in tip-top condition. It will also help to strengthen the hair and stimulate growth, and keep the scalp clean and fresh. To be effective, a tonic should be used regularly and massaged gently into the scalp.

Recommended herbs for hair tonics

Burdock	Fennel	Lime flowers
Catnip	Horsetail	Nettle
Cleavers	Lavender	Rosemary

Take 30 g (1 tblsp) fresh or 10 g (1 tsp) dried of your chosen herb(s) (you can use a combination, choosing from the list above) and pour on 150 ml (1 cup) boiling water (double these amounts for long hair). Leave for 30 minutes, then filter and cool. Add the juice of one lemon and 20 ml (1 tblsp) cider vinegar. Apply as a final rinse after shampooing the hair, massaging the scalp. Then lightly rinse off, using a minimal amount of cool water.

Enhancing natural colour

Natural herbal dyes to colour and lighten the hair have been used for hundreds of years, and they do not contain the harsh chemicals of many over-the-counter products which can often leave locks damaged and weakened.

When using natural herbal colorants, the results are more unpredictable than the achievable shades which match the colours given on the guide charts of commercially sold tints and dyes. So it's advisable to do a strand test on a piece of hair that's hidden, such as behind your ears, to get an idea of the overall effect. Start off cautiously – use a weak version of your chosen herbal colorant and build up gradually to your desired shade. This is better than using too much straight away and being stuck with the results. Always wear rubber gloves to protect your hands when applying herbal colorants.

Recommended herbs for colour enhancers

Blonde/ fair hair	Dark hair	Red hair	Grey hair
Chamomile	Elderflower	Marigold	Elderflower
St John's wort	Rosemary		Sage
	Sage		

Make a strong decoction simmering 60g (2 tblsp) fresh or 20g (2 tsp) dried of your chosen herb in a litre water for 20 minutes in a covered pan. Cool, strain and pour the filtered liquid through the hair catching the rinse in a bowl. Repeat several times, then pat hair dry with an old towel. For a more intense colour, make the rinse into a paste. Use 150ml (1 cup) of water for the decoction and 30g (1 tblsp) fresh or 10g (1 tsp) dried herb. Boil for 10 minutes, cool and strain. Then add enough kaolin powder to make a smooth paste. Apply to the hair roots gradually working down the strands of the hair. Cover the hair with a small plastic bag and then a hot towel. Leave on for 20 minutes and then rinse off thoroughly. Several applications may be necessary to achieve the desired shade.

Sage and tea darkening decoction

This combination is ideal for masking premature greying hair. You will need:

- 20g (2 tsp) dried sage
- 20g (2 tsp) tea-leaves
- 500ml still mineral water
- 10ml (2 tsp) vodka

Put the sage and tea in a pan and add the water. Bring to the boil, cover and simmer over a gentle heat for about two hours. Remove from heat and cool. Strain and stir in vodka. Bottle and store in fridge. Rub this decoction into the scalp five times a week to help mask premature greying of the hair.

Chamomile blonde highlighter

You will need:

- 375ml still mineral water
- 150g (5 tblsp) fresh or 50g (5 tsp) dried chamomile flowers
- 240g (8 tblsp) kaolin powder
- 1 egg yolk, beaten

Heat the water and, when boiling, pour over the chamomile flowers and simmer for 25 minutes. Cool and then strain off 250ml of liquid. Gradually add enough of the liquid to the kaolin to mix to a smooth paste. Stir in the rest of the liquid a little at a time until thoroughly blended. Add the egg yolk and mix well. Apply to the hair and leave on for 20–50 minutes. Rinse off thoroughly with warm water. Several applications may be needed to lighten natural fair tones.

Herbal hair treats

Herbal warm oil repair treatment
Hair that lacks lustre and is prone to dryness and split ends should be treated to a warm herbal oil treatment once a month before a shampoo. This will help to replenish valuable lost moisture and correct any dryness. Apply your herbal oil and then relax in a warm bath, the added warmth is ideal for this treatment.

Recommended herbs	
Burdock	Nettle
Marshmallow	Parsley

Make an infused herbal oil (see Preparing Herbs, page 17) using one of the recommended herbs. For your hair treatment simply warm the oil gently, pour a little into the palm of your hand and rub your hands together. Gently massage onto the hair and scalp, paying particular attention to the hair ends. Cover your hair with foil or a shower cap and then wrap in a hot towel. (The best way to heat a towel is to dip it in hot water then wring it out.) Leave for 20–30 minutes, replacing the towel as it cools. Wash off with shampoo and rinse thoroughly.

Minty-fresh hair rinse

This peppermint rinse will not only get rid of any last traces of soapy residue which can leave the hair looking dull and the scalp dry and scaly, it will also help restore the acidic balance of the hair often stripped by modern, proprietary shampoos. You will need:

- 240g (8 tblsp) fresh peppermint leaves, chopped
- 1 litre still mineral water
- 1 litre cider vinegar

Bring the peppermint leaves to the boil in the water, cover and simmer for 10 minutes. Remove from heat and allow to infuse for one hour. Strain and stir in the cider vinegar. Bottle and leave for 48 hours before use. After washing your hair, add 500ml to the final rinse water. Store in the fridge and use within one week.

Rosemary pre-wash conditioner

An enriching treatment for your hair if you've been under the weather and your hair's suffered, or a perfect holiday hair repair conditioner when the sun, salty sea water or heavily chlorinated swimming pool water have left it weakened and dry. As well as restoring body and bounce, rosemary is superb for putting the lustre and life back into your locks! You will need:

- 40ml (2 tblsp) avocado oil
- 20ml (1 tblsp) castor oil
- 10ml (2 tsp) rosemary infusion
- 2 eggs

Whisk all the ingredients together until the mixture is light and airy. Then, using the fingertips, massage the conditioner evenly through the hair and into the scalp. Wrap the hair in a towel and leave for 20 minutes and then shampoo and rinse in the normal way. Make fresh for each application.

Yogurt and lime flowers flyaway hair formula
A great conditioner for fine, flyaway hair. You will need:

- 120ml (6 tblsp) natural yogurt
- 1 egg, beaten
- 40ml (2 tblsp) standard infusion of lime flowers

Whisk the yogurt and egg together until thoroughly blended. Gradually stir in the infusion of lime flowers. After shampooing and rinsing out the hair, towel dry. Massage the conditioner evenly into the hair and scalp, wrap in a warm towel and leave for 10–15 minutes. Rinse out thoroughly with lukewarm water. Make fresh for each application.

THE BODY

Along with the face and hair, the rest of the body should not miss out on its fair share of care and attention in order to keep it looking good. The hands and feet in particular suffer a lot of wear and tear and are often subjected to extremes of temperature and need to be pampered accordingly. But the rest of the body can also benefit greatly from regular restorative treatments.

Dull-looking skin and the build-up of cellulite is often down to poor circulation. Regular exercise and a healthy diet with plenty of fresh fruit and vegetables goes a long way to help prevent the build-up of toxins, allowing the blood to flow freely, which in turn makes the skin appear glowing and healthy-looking. But stimulating body treatments, using simple-to-make herbal preparations, can also improve overall skin tone and help you achieve the body beautiful.

Herbal bath infusions

An aromatic herbal bath is one of the most pleasurable and therapeutic of body treatments. Certain herbs will revive and rejuvenate, stimulating the circulation. Some help soothe and relax both the mind and body ready for a good night's sleep, while other herbs can simply be enjoyed for their wonderful fragrance.

Recommended herbs

Relaxing	Reviving	Relieves tired/ aching muscles
Basil	Alehoof (ground ivy)	Angelica
Catnip	Elderflower	Fennel
Chamomile	Fennel	Horsetail
Cowslip flowers	Hyssop	Lady's mantle
Lavender	Lemon balm	Marigold
Lime flowers	Peppermint	Sage
Marshmallow	Rosemary	Yarrow
Valerian	Sage	
Vervain	Thyme	

Fill small, home-made bags made from squares of muslin or cheesecloth with your chosen herb(s) (you can use a combination from your selected group) and hang over the hot water stream as you run your bath. Alternatively, you could use three or four shop-bought herbal 'teabags', or simply infuse a handful of your chosen herb(s) in 1½ litres of boiling water, strain, and add to your bath. Another alternative is to make up a herbal infused oil or tincture (see Preparing Herbs, page 17) and add 10 drops of this to your bath once it has run. Then mix it around with your hand. Don't add home-made herbal infused oil directly to hot running water as it will evaporate.

Skin softening milk bath

Add milk to your herbal bath infusion to leave your skin feeling silky smooth. Add 60g (2 tblsp) powdered milk (not skimmed as it doesn't have the same effect) to a fine gauze or muslin bag along with 60g (2 tblsp) fresh or 30g (1 tblsp) dried of any one (or a combination) of the following finely chopped herbs: elderflowers, chamomile flowers or lime flowers. Then hang the bag over the hot tap as you run the bath water. Alternatively, infuse 45g (1½ tblsp) of the fresh flowers in 250ml of fresh, cold milk for two hours. Strain and then add to the bath. If using fresh milk, make up fresh for each bath.

Herbal massage oil

Make a herbal infused oil (see Preparing Herbs, page 17) using the recommended herb of your choice and use for either an uplifting, relaxing or soothing body massage.

Herbal body treats

Herbal body buffer

A daily body toning scrub will help kickstart the circulation and eliminate toxins via the lymphatic system, so helping to break down the fatty deposits which lead to the build-up of cellulite. Simply add a little fine oatmeal or bran to your home-made herbal muslin bags and rub all over the body, or make up the following body booster. You will need:

- 90g (3 tblsp) fine sea salt or fine oatmeal
- 1 ripe avocado, mashed to a pulp
- juice of 1 lemon
- 40ml (2 tblsp) of the herbal infusion of your choice

Mix all the ingredients together, then rub vigorously over the body using a hemp mitt, loofah or natural bristle brush. With long, sweeping movements, start at the feet and work up the legs and across the hips and bottom, also up the arms, upper back and gently across the chest and stomach. Then shower off thoroughly with warm water.

Herbal all-over body tonic
Makes an ideal body toner to tighten pores after a shower or bath. You will need:

- 10g (1 tsp) of either dried meadowsweet, nettle, witch hazel or star anise seed
- 75ml (½ cup) of boiling water
- 20ml (1 tblsp) glycerine

Steep the chosen herb in the boiling water. Allow to cool, then strain and leave to stand for 30 minutes. Add the glycerine and mix thoroughly. Apply a little on a cotton wool pad to the whole body after a shower or bath to tone up the skin. Store in the fridge and use within three days.

Ivy anti-cellulite cream
A cream that will hit the problem spots and help break down the fatty deposits that accumulate to form cellulite. You will need:

- 20g (2 tsp) finely chopped fresh or dried common ivy
- 20ml (1 tblsp) sunflower oil
- ground almonds or fine oatmeal

Warm the ivy in the sunflower oil. Remove from heat and stir in enough ground almonds or oatmeal to make a paste. Massage this mixture into the problem areas firmly, using strong circular movements and then rinse off with warm water. Make up fresh for each application.

HANDS

It's important to protect your hands to keep them soft and in good condition. Cold weather, sunlight and soapy detergents can all take their toll, leaving hands dry and rough. So why not keep your favourite herbal preparation by the sink so that every time you wash your hands, your herbal remedy is ready to apply.

Herbal hand infusion
Soaking the hands in a warm standard infusion made from any one (or a combination) of the following herbs will help keep them soft and smooth. Choose from: chamomile, fennel, lady's mantle, marigold, marshmallow or yarrow.

Herbal hand treats

Marigold and oatmeal hand cleanser
This natural cleanser leaves hands beautifully clean and soft. Pour a little fine oatmeal into the palm of one hand. Add sufficient standard infusion of marigold just to moisten it. Massage the oatmeal into the hands and then rinse off with warm water.

Marigold hand cream
You will need:

- 30g (1 tblsp) fresh or 10g (1 tsp) dried marigold flowers
- 125ml boiling water
- 15g (½ tblsp) cornflour
- 20ml (1 tblsp) sunflower oil
- 3ml (½ tsp) honey

Add the marigold flowers to the boiling water and leave to infuse for 30 minutes, then strain. Mix the cornflour and the sunflower oil into a smooth paste. Over a gentle heat, dissolve the honey in the strained infusion and blend well, then remove from heat and gradually add to the paste. Return to a gentle heat and bring to boiling point, stirring continuously. Remove from the heat and when cooled, pour into a screwtop container. Massage into the hands as required. Store in the fridge and use within four days.

Marshmallow rough skin saver

Soak 30g (1 tblsp) grated dried marshmallow root in 150ml (1 cup) of cold water for about eight hours. Strain, then heat the liquid by placing it in a bowl over a pan of hot water until lukewarm, stirring continuously until the liquid thickens slightly. Add this marshmallow extract to 20ml (1 tblsp) of glycerine and mix thoroughly. Pour into a screwtop jar. Massage a little into the hands at night to soften rough skin and chapped hands. Use within four days.

Lady's mantle hand conditioner

Once a week, treat your hands to a rich moisturising treatment. You will need:

- 30g (1 tblsp) fine oatmeal
- 10ml (½ tblsp) standard infusion of lady's mantle
- 3ml (½ tsp) avocado oil

- 3 ml (½ tsp) lemon juice
- 3 ml (½ tsp) glycerine

Mix the ingredients together to form a paste. Dampen the hands with a little warm water and rub a small amount of the conditioner onto the hands thoroughly. Then, using the sides of the first finger and the thumb, massage each finger one by one. Always work from the nail end towards the hand. Now massage with the thumb in between the fingers and with the thumb tip massage each nail, working in the cream. Repeat these massage techniques on the other hand. Leave for 20 minutes and then rinse with lukewarm water. Use fresh for each application.

Horsetail nail strengthener
You will need:

- 10 g (1 tsp) fresh horsetail leaves, finely chopped
- 75 ml (½ cup) boiling water
- 20 ml (1 tblsp) honey

Steep the horsetail in the boiling water and leave for 30 minutes. Strain. Take 5 ml (1 tsp) of the infusion and add the honey. Mix well. Soak nails in this mixture for 5–10 minutes. Rinse with lukewarm water, dry gently and then apply hand cream. Use fresh for each application. The horsetail infusion can be stored in the fridge for two to three days.

FEET

Like your hands, your feet need proper care and attention to keep them feeling and looking good. In fact most common problems are caused by neglect or worse by squashing them into ill-fitting shoes or boots. So treat your feet to some herbal remedies and you'll soon be walking on air!

Recommended herbs for the feet

Refreshing	*Deodorising*	*Soothing*
Lavender	Angelica	Chamomile
Lime flowers	Rosemary	Elderflower
Marigold	Sage	Horsetail
Nettle		Lavender
Peppermint		Marigold
Rosemary		Peppermint
Thyme		Thyme

Herbal footbath

Fill a large bowl or half fill a bath with very hot water. Add 30g (1 tblsp) fresh or 10g (1 tsp) dried of the herb(s) of your choice (you can use a combination of herbs from your selected group). Add 60g (2 tblsp) sea salt or 30g (1 tblsp) Epsom salts. Leave with a towel over the top until the water has cooled sufficiently to be bearable for the feet. Sit and soak for 10 minutes. Rinse the feet, dry gently and then apply a moisturising cream.

Herbal feet treats

Marigold and lime foot lotion

Relieve hot, aching feet with this revitalising foot lotion. You will need:

- 40 ml (2 tblsp) standard infusion of marigold
- 5 ml (1 tsp) lime juice
- 5 ml (1 tsp) rose water

Mix all the ingredients together. Soak your hands in the lotion and massage the feet. Store in the fridge and use within a week.

Lavender foot oil
A rich moisturising alternative to the foot lotion. Massage after soaking in a foot bath. You will need:

- 60 ml (3 tblsp) sunflower oil
- 10 ml (½ tblsp) cider vinegar
- 5 drops of lavender herbal oil
- 5 g (½ tsp) alum powder (available from chemists or health food shops)

Put all the ingredients into a bowl over a pan of hot water and heat gently, stirring continuously. Remove from heat and allow to cool, then pour into a sterilized jam jar, screw on the lid and shake thoroughly. Remove the lid until completely cold. Shake again before use. Massage a small amount of the oil into the feet. Use within three days.

Peppermint foot balm
A moisturising balm that softens hard skin and callouses on the feet. You will need:

- 20 ml (1 tblsp) standard infusion of marigold
- 30 g (1 tblsp) vegetable fat, softened
- 4 drops of oil of peppermint

Carefully blend the marigold infusion with the softened vegetable fat in a bowl. Add the drops of peppermint oil and blend well. Spoon into a screwtop glass container. Massage a little into the feet after a herbal foot soak. Keep in the fridge and use within two weeks.

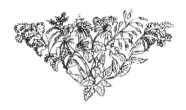

4

Herbs for health

The use of herbs for their healing and curative properties can be found in the history of all races – it is as old as humanity itself. And yet this form of medicine, whose majority of remedies have been in use for thousands of years, is considered 'alternative' while the modern man-made pharmaceuticals developed by the Western world are deemed 'orthodox'.

Despite the advent of sophisticated drugs, traditional plant remedies still provide about 85 per cent of the world's medicines. And not just in the poorer developing countries, where the cost of modern drugs make them prohibitive. With the growing anxiety over the numerous side effects of today's synthetic drugs, more and more people are looking for more natural, safe and effective forms of medication, such as herbs, to help them take greater responsibility for their own health.

Unlike many modern medicines, which simply aim to alleviate the *symptoms* of a particular condition, herbal medicine takes an holistic approach to illness in that it aims to treat the *cause* of the problem and therefore help the body as a whole. For example, a fever is one of the ways the body fights off infection. Just to get rid of the fever, not only does nothing to deal with the infection but it also suppresses the body's own defences. Herbalism, however, aims to support and enhance these natural defence mechanisms and stimulate the body's own responses to heal the condition effectively.

Herbal medicines, however, cannot provide any miracle cures. Looking after your body by eating a well-balanced diet, making sure you get plenty of sleep, taking regular exercise and having sufficient relaxation provides the best foundation for promoting healing which is vital if the herbal remedies are to prove fully effective. Actually including fresh herbs, which contain many valuable trace elements, minerals and vitamins in your diet can also help boost the body's immune system.

The plants featured in this chapter are a selection of the more easily available herbs that may safely be used following the given recommendations to treat a wide variety of common ailments at home. However, such self-help treatments should only be used for mild infections and conditions. For more serious complaints always consult a doctor or a qualified herbal practitioner.

It should never be forgotten that herbs are also potent drugs. Remedies should not be taken long term, and the recommended dosage should never be exceeded. If symptoms persist or the condition worsens, consult your doctor. Some herbs can interact with orthodox drugs so if you suffer from a persistent medical condition and are already taking medication for a particular complaint, always consult your GP or a qualified herbalist before taking any herbal remedies.

In this chapter, a selection of common ailments – together with their suggested herbal remedies – are listed in alphabetical order. Associated conditions included elsewhere in the chapter, which may be appropriate when considering treatment, are given in bold for easy reference underneath the entry heading.

For each ailment, a number of herbal remedies are given

and the choice of which remedy to use will depend on the availability of the herb and its particular relevance to the symptoms of the sufferer.

All remedies in this chapter are based on standard quantities of herbs, as given in Chapter 2, Preparing Herbs (see pages 11–19) unless stated otherwise. When using a combination of herbs, the total amount should not exceed the standard recommended quantity.

The standard recommended adult dosage for each method, where appropriate, is as follows:

INFUSION	One teacup three times a day, unless otherwise stated.
DECOCTION	One teacup three times a day, unless otherwise stated.
TINCTURE	5 ml (1 tsp) diluted in a little water three times a day, unless otherwise stated.

Before preparing any medicinal remedy, always look up the particular herb you want to use in Chapter 5, The A–Z of Herbs (see pages 97–140) for a complete plant profile and take note of any cautions. Then refer to Chapter 2, Preparing Herbs (see pages 11–19) for how to prepare your chosen herb for use in the remedy.

Many home-made herbal remedies do not keep for long periods, so it is best to make up these preparations fresh for each application, rather than to prepare large quantities and store them. Make sure all storage bottles and containers are clean and thoroughly sterilised in boiling water before use. Keep in the fridge, away from food, unless specified. Don't forget to label and date each remedy.

Note
For children under four, only give one quarter of the standard adult dose; for children between the ages of four and seven and for adults over 70 or for those who are frail or convalescing, use half the standard adult dose. When treating children between the ages of seven and 12 years, give three quarters of the adult dose.

Herbal first aid

There are a number of herbal remedies (those which have a reasonable shelf life) that can be added to your first aid kit at home, so they are ready to use whenever you need them. Recommendations include: herbal infused lavender oil to repel insects; antiseptic and antibacterial marigold ointment for cuts, grazes and wounds; distilled witch hazel for minor burns, bruises, sprains, wasp stings and mosquito bites; tincture of yarrow to stop bleeding of minor cuts and wounds; and tincture of myrrh for an antiseptic gargle. See Chapter 2, Preparing Herbs (pages 11–19) for instructions on how to make these remedies.

Acid stomach
(see also **indigestion**)

This usually refers to the regurgitation of acid or partly digested food from the stomach into the oesophagus (food pipe) or mouth. This can be caused by over-eating or drinking, or bending down or exertion too soon after eating. In some cases the condition can indicate a more serious complaint, so if symptoms persist, see a doctor.

Herbal remedies
- A standard infusion of marshmallow (if using the root, make a standard decoction) will help reduce irritation of the stomach, or a standard infusion of meadowsweet will reduce excess stomach acid.
- A standard infusion of yarrow or 10g (1 tsp) of slippery elm powder dissolved in 150ml (1 cup) of hot water will help tone and heal the digestive system.
- A cup of standard infusion of chamomile taken before a meal will help settle the stomach and act as a digestive

tonic. Sweeten with 5 ml (1 tsp) honey if desired.

- One hour before a meal, take 10–15 drops of tincture of angelica diluted in 150 ml (1 cup) of water, to help reduce acidity.

Acne and spots
(see also **boils and sores**)

Acne – the inflammation of the sebaceous glands on the face, chest and back causing spots and pimples – is most likely to occur during adolescence due to the hormonal changes taking place. But diet can also be a factor. Avoid fatty, sugary foods, dairy produce and chocolate and eat plenty of fresh fruit and vegetables.

Herbal remedies
- A facial steam helps open pores which have become blocked and reduces any inflammation and infection. Use 30 g (1 tblsp) of fresh or 10 g (1 tsp) dried of any one (or a combination) of the following herbs: chamomile, sage or yarrow. Place chosen herbs in a bowl and pour over enough boiling water to half fill the bowl. Bend your face over the bowl for five minutes, covering your head and the bowl with a towel to trap in the steam. Then gently wipe face with cotton wool.
- For an anti-bacterial skinwash, cleanse affected area daily with a standard infusion made from any combination of the following: chamomile, which is purifying; lavender, calming and slightly antiseptic; marigold, which is antiseptic and antibacterial; and thyme, which is also a strong germ-killer.
- To cleanse the skin from within, take a standard herbal infusion made from any one of the following herbs: burdock, cleavers or echinacea (a herbal antibiotic).

- Make up a herbal compress using herb Robert, a herbal astringent, and apply to the affected area.
- To bring the spots to a head, apply a drawing paste. Mix equal amounts of grated dried marshmallow root and slippery elm powder with enough water to make a stiff paste. Apply over the affected area and leave on for at least 20 minutes (or overnight) before rinsing off gently with tepid water.
- Apply an ointment made with marigold flowers at night to soothe and heal.

Anaemia

Anaemia – a deficiency of the oxygen-carrying substance haemoglobin in the red blood cells – has a variety of causes. One of the most common is a lack of iron, one of the trace elements vital to the production of red blood cells. If this is the case then make sure your diet includes plenty of iron-rich foods which include green vegetables such as spinach plus nettles, parsley, dried apricots and fish.

Herbal remedies
- Take a cup of standard warm infusion made using either nettle or parsley, both iron-rich herbs, three times a day.

Arthritis
(see also **rheumatism**)

This is a widespread term for a variety of different conditions all involving some kind of swelling, pain or stiffness of the joints. The two most common types are osteoarthritis and rheumatoid arthritis. Whatever the type of arthritis you are treating, a balanced, wholefood diet is

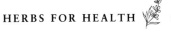

also essential. Some foods such as red meat and some citrus fruits such as oranges can aggravate the condition.

Herbal remedies

- A standard infusion using any one (or a combination) of the following herbs will help clear waste products which can accumulate around the joints and lead to inflammation. Choose from burdock, dandelion, meadowsweet or parsley.
- To improve circulation, take a standard infusion of hawthorn.
- Arthritis can be triggered by severe stress and anxiety. Help relieve pain and relax the nervous system with a standard infusion of valerian.

Asthma

There are several herbs which can help this condition, in which the small bronchial airways temporarily constrict, making it difficult to breathe and causing a wheezing sound as the breath is exhaled. Severe asthma can be life threatening and requires professional medical help. Chronic sufferers should consult their doctor or a qualified medical practitioner before taking herbal remedies.

Herbal remedies

- Soak the root of elecampane in water for about 8–10 hours. Then add 30g (1 tblsp) of soaked root to 500ml of water, bring to boiling point and allow to cool and then strain. Drink one cup of this infusion three times a day to help the lungs and loosen mucus.
- A warm standard infusion using either white horehound or thyme will make a useful expectorant and antispasmodic to help relax the muscles to aid breathing.

- A cup of a standard infusion made with 30g (1 tblsp) fresh, finely chopped fennel leaves or crushed seeds and 150ml (1 cup) of boiling water will help clear the bronchial tubes and soothe coughing.

Athlete's foot

This fungal infection is most commonly found between the toes but can affect any area of the skin. It is highly contagious especially in warm, moist conditions. To prevent the spread of infection use separate towels and always wash your hands after touching infected areas.

Herbal remedies
- Bathe feet in a footbath made from a standard infusion using a combination of agrimony, marigold and sage plus 10ml (2 tsp) of cider vinegar. Soak for about 30 minutes then dry carefully.
- To help fight the infection and boost the immune system, make a standard infusion using a combination of burdock, dandelion leaves, echinacea, nettle and peppermint. Drink one cup three times a day.
- Apply an ointment made with marigold flowers to soothe irritation and destroy the infection.

Bad breath

Eating strongly flavoured and spicy food can cause bad breath, but if the condition persists it could be a sign of poor digestion, that the teeth are in need of attention or the gums are infected and a dentist or doctor should be consulted.

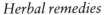

Herbal remedies

- Chew fresh, washed aniseed or parsley leaves to neutral-ise strong odours on the breath, such as garlic. Parsley has a high chlorophyll content, and this green pigment is used in many commercially made breath fresheners.
- Make a standard infusion of peppermint and either drink or use as a refreshing mouthwash.
- Chewing raw or crystallised ginger will sweeten the breath.

Baldness

Although shedding hair is a natural process, sometimes due to severe shock, stress or prolonged illness, the hair can suddenly start to fall out in large clumps. If this is the case, it is best to see your doctor immediately. Once the underlying cause has been treated, the hair usually returns to normal within a few months. Most cases of baldness, however, do not happen so quickly. Gradually the shed hair fails to regrow resulting in a bald patch that gets bigger and bigger over the years. This type of baldness is usually hereditary but can be helped by a number of herbal remedies to help stimulate growth.

Herbal remedies

- Nettle is an excellent hair conditioner with a reputation for helping prevent hair loss. Using gloves, place a large handful of fresh nettles in a pan with enough cold water to cover. Bring to the boil, cover and simmer for 15 minutes. Strain the liquid and cool. Use as a final rinse after shampooing, or massage gently into the scalp and comb through hair.
- An infusion made with chamomile will help stimulate growth and leave hair soft and shining. Pour 600ml

(4 cups) of boiling water on 90g (3 tblsp) fresh or 30g (1 tblsp) dried chamomile flowers. Leave to stand for two hours. Strain and reheat until gently warm and rinse over hair several times after shampooing, massaging well into the scalp.

Bites and stings

Some people suffer severe allergic reactions to insect bites and stings. If this is the case, seek expert advice immediately.

Herbal remedies
- When bees sting they leave their stings behind in the skin which must then be removed. Use a pair of tweezers, sterilised in boiling water. Bee stings are acid and should be neutralised by applying a little sodium bicarbonate, mixed into a paste with a little water, to the affected area.
- Wasp stings are alkaline. For wasp stings and mosquito bites, apply a little neat lemon juice or distilled witch hazel or a slice of raw onion.
- Lavender infused herbal oil will help repel insects and also help relieve discomfort.
- Rub fresh basil or plantain (plantago major) leaves on insect bites to ease itching and inflammation.
- Drink one cup of a standard infusion made with echinacea, a herbal antibiotic, three times a day.
- An ointment made with soothing marshmallow leaf applied to the sting or bite will help relieve discomfort.

Blood pressure (low and high)

Any fluctuation in blood pressure should always be monitored by a qualified expert. But there are steps you can take yourself to help your condition. Low blood pressure only becomes a problem when it is accompanied by circulation difficulties, dizziness or fainting. The most common causes of high blood pressure, or hypertension, are stress, obesity or the hardening of the arteries leading from the heart. A diet high in fresh fruit and vegetables and wholegrain cereals, that avoids red meat, salt which causes fluid retention, and stimulants such as tea and coffee will help the condition. Regular exercise and relaxation are also important.

Herbal remedies
- For low blood pressure, herbs that help to boost the circulation include ginger and oats. Take ginger as a standard infusion. Oats can either be prepared with a little water and taken as porridge or as a tincture. To make the tincture, grind oats up coarsely and add one part oats to two parts of alcohol. Then dilute this with water equal to the amount of alcohol used. Pour into an airtight container and leave for two weeks, shaking once a day. Then strain and take 20 ml (1 tblsp) morning and evening.
- A standard infusion of rosemary acts as a general tonic for the circulatory system, especially beneficial to those who suffer from low blood pressure and who tire easily.
- If your blood pressure is high, a standard infusion of hawthorn combined with lime flowers and/or yarrow will help lower it.
- Add valerian to the above infusion if you suffer from stress.
- Eating raw garlic benefits the circulation and it can also

Note
Do consult your doctor or a qualified herbal practitioner before taking herbal remedies for a heart condition.

help lower blood cholesterol, a fatty deposit that can cause a hardening of the arteries which supply the heart.

- If you suffer from high blood pressure it's important to avoid a build-up of excess fluid in the body. To lessen any fluid retention avoid adding salt to your food, which promotes water retention. Also a standard infusion of dandelion leaves, a good diuretic herb, will help relieve any fluid build-up. Alternatively, during the spring and summer months add fresh, washed dandelion leaves to salads.
- To ease stress a relaxing herbal bath using lavender or lemon balm will also help you unwind.

Boils and sores
(see also acne and spots)

Boils and sores – painful, inflamed swellings – often occur when there is a build-up of impurities within the body or when the body is run-down.

Herbal remedies
- Blood-cleansing herbs, such as burdock and echinacea, will help rid the system of impurities. Use 30g (1 tblsp) fresh or 10g (1 tsp) of dried finely chopped herb to 150ml (1 cup) of boiling water and when cool, strain and take 20ml (1 tblsp) every two to three hours.
- Take raw garlic to fight any infection.
- Apply a hot poultice to the affected area to draw out the impurities using astringent plantain (plantago major) leaves or antibacterial marigold flowers.
- Alternatively use a herbal drawing out powder. Mix equal parts of grated dried marshmallow root and slippery elm powder into a thick paste with a little

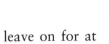

water. Apply to the affected area and leave on for at least 20 minutes (or overnight) before gently rinsing off with tepid water.

Bronchitis
(see also **catarrh, coughs**)

The bronchial tubes become inflamed and painful, causing thick catarrh accompanied by a wheezing cough.

Herbal remedies
- A standard infusion of a herb with an expectorant action such as white horehound or thyme will help loosen the phlegm and bring relief. Or infuse 10g (1 tsp) of shredded elecampane root in 150ml (1 cup) of cold water for nine hours. Strain and then reheat liquid and drink while hot. Add echinacea to your chosen infusion to boost the immune system and help fight the infection.
- Eating cloves of raw garlic will also help fight the infection.
- A standard infusion of hyssop, which is also an expectorant herb, or angelica, a warming antiseptic, is also beneficial for chest complaints.
- To bring down a fever, cool the body and help clear the infection, take a standard infusion using either elderflowers, yarrow or lime flowers.
- Mix 4–5 drops of peppermint essential oil, which contains menthol, an antibacterial, with 20ml (4 tsp) soya oil and use in an inhalation to help clear the bronchial airways.

Bruises

A bruise occurs when skin tissue is injured. If a bruise doesn't fade after about a week or if one appears after only a minor injury, consult your doctor.

Herbal remedies
- To reduce the pain and swelling of a bruise, apply a cold compress made with a standard infusion of marigold or witch hazel leaves or a standard decoction if using witch hazel bark.
- Alternatively, make up herbal ice cubes by pouring your preferred infusion, once cooled, into an ice tray and freeze. Then apply to the bruise.
- Boil fresh burdock or herb Robert leaves in salt water for a few minutes and apply as a poultice to the bruise to help reduce any inflammation.

Burns

For severe burns summon professional help immediately, meanwhile cool burn with cool (not ice cold) water but do not remove any clothing that is stuck to the wound. For minor burns and scolds immerse the affected area in cold water immediately for about 5–10 minutes until the pain subsides.

Herbal remedies
- To soothe and relieve pain, apply a compress of distilled witch hazel or a cooled standard infusion of either chamomile or marigold. This will also speed healing and minimise blistering depending on the severity of the burn.
- Once the pain has lessened, cover loosely with a dry, sterile, non-fluffy dressing.

Catarrh
(see also **bronchitis, coughs, colds, earache, hay fever**)

Catarrh – where the lining of the airways becomes inflamed causing an increase in the amount of mucus discharged, which then accumulates in the nose or on the chest – often accompanies a cold or can be caused by an allergy to pollen or dust such as hay fever. To ease the condition, avoid all milk and dairy products, reduce carbohydrates and eat plenty of fresh fruit and vegetables.

Herbal remedies
- A standard infusion of any combination of the following expectorant herbs will help loosen and expel thick catarrh: alehoof (ground ivy), elecampane, eyebright, fennel leaves, white horehound, hyssop or thyme. Or try a standard decoction of cowslip root. Add echinacea to the above infusions or decoction to fight any infection.
- An inhalation using chamomile, peppermint or thyme, once or twice a week, will help clear the airways.
- Mix 15 drops of eucalyptus oil with 50ml (2½ tblsp) soya oil and massage the front of the chest and back and between the shoulder blades twice a day.
- Herbs that specifically tone mucus membrane that has suffered from catarrh include alehoof (ground ivy) and plantain (plantago lanceolata). Take either herb as a standard infusion.

Colds
(see also **bronchitis, catarrh, coughs, fever, sore throat**)

Herbs can be used in the effective treatment of colds by supporting and improving the function of the immune system, and repelling hostile viruses and bacteria. To prevent and treat colds, make sure your diet is rich in vitamin C and garlic to fight off infection.

Herbal remedies
- At the first signs of a cold, drink a cup of the following warm infusion, made with diaphoretic herbs (herbs that promote sweating) twice a day. Put 5g (½ tsp) each of dried catnip, elderflowers, peppermint and yarrow into a bowl. Pour over 250ml of boiling water. Leave to stand for one minute, strain and then add 5ml (1 tsp) of honey and a pinch of cayenne pepper. Keep in fridge and reheat as necessary.
- A standard infusion using any one (or a combination) of the following herbs is also beneficial: aniseed, ginger and white horehound – all warming expectorant and tonic herbs; catnip to help bring down a fever; eyebright for nasal congestion; angelica or sage to fight infection.
- A steam inhalation will help clear the nose and throat. Pour boiling water over 10g (1 tsp) of each of the following dried herbs: chamomile, nettle, peppermint or thyme.

Colitis
(see also **diarrhoea**)

Colitis – inflammation or irritation of the large intestine – which causes diarrhoea, sometimes with blood, abdominal pain and possibly fever, may be due to infection, high levels of stress or sometimes food intolerance. It's always worth omitting foods such as tea, coffee, milk products and eggs from the diet on a temporary basis and noting the effect.

Note
If symptoms persist, consult your doctor.

Herbal remedies
- Dissolve 10g (1 tsp) of slippery elm powder into 150ml

(1 cup) of hot water and drink to soothe the irritated colon. Repeat twice a day.

- Alternatively, a standard decoction of marshmallow root, which produces a protective mucilage (gel-like substance) will help soothe the intestine.
- If suffering from high anxiety and tension, a calming cup of a standard infusion made with chamomile and valerian, both natural herbal relaxants, will help soothe, or try a cup of standard infusion of agrimony, a mild astringent, which will treat the infection.

Conjunctivitis

This condition arises when the transparent membrane, the conjunctiva, that covers the white of the eye and inside the lids, becomes irritated and inflamed, causing redness and pain. Sometimes the eye is left sticky and crusted, especially after a night's sleep. Conjunctivitis is usually caused by an infection or an allergy such as hay fever or exposure to pollution in the atmosphere.

Herbal remedies
- Using a separate, sterilised eyebath for each eye, bathe with a standard cooled decoction of either agrimony, chamomile, chickweed, elderflowers, eyebright, marigold or plantain (plantago major).
- Alternatively, make up a standard decoction using herb Robert, marigold, vervain or witch hazel and apply as a compress to soothe the eyes. Use a separate compress for each eye.
- Drinking a cup of a standard infusion made with a combination of burdock, cleavers, echinacea, horsetail and antiseptic and anti-inflammatory eyebright three times a day boosts the immune system to help fight infection.

Note
All herbal solutions applied to the eye must be thoroughly strained three times through fine muslin cloth or a jelly bag before being used, in order to prevent any small particles entering the eye and causing further pain, irritation or even infection. For all external herbal eye remedies, always simmer herbs in boiling water for at least 10 minutes to make sure they are thoroughly sterilised.

Constipation

Constipation is caused by a lack of regular action of the bowel, so the body fails to get rid of its waste. This is often caused by a diet lacking in fibre, a lack of exercise and/or high levels of stress and anxiety. To help correct the condition it's important to include fibre in your diet to aid digestion and promote a healthy bowel action. Raw bran, whilst being a rich source of fibre, can interfere with the absorption of key minerals such as iron, calcium and magnesium, instead eat plenty of fibre-rich foods such as fruit, vegetables and wholegrain bread and cereals. Prunes are known to help ease the condition but there are also some herbs known for their natural, gentle laxative action.

Note
Such remedies should only be used as a short-term solution. If the problem persists consult a doctor.

Herbal remedies

- A cup, once or twice a day, of a standard decoction made from ginger and dandelion root makes a gentle but effective herbal laxative. A standard infusion of fumitory will help a sluggish digestion. Add chamomile if suffering from tension or stress.

Coughs
(see also **bronchitis, catarrh, colds, fever, sore throat**)

The best way to treat a cough is to get rid of what is causing it, rather than just suppressing it. The action of coughing itself is the body's way of expelling congested mucus or inhaled dust from the lungs, bronchial tubes or windpipe. Causes vary from an irritant through to an infection.

Herbal remedies

- A cup of a hot standard infusion of white horehound or a standard decoction made with cowslip root, three times a day, will help dispel mucus from the lungs and alleviate a dry cough.

- For an irritating, dry cough a standard infusion of marshmallow leaves to soothe the throat and chest combines well with white horehound.
- For catarrhal coughs, a standard infusion using a combination of expectorant, antibiotic herbs such as elecampane, elderflowers, hyssop and thyme will help alleviate the condition.
- For a cough with a fever, take a standard infusion of angelica or yarrow.
- For lingering coughs, take a standard infusion using any one (or a combination) of the following: hyssop, marshmallow leaves or thyme.
- To help fight bronchial infections, a clove of raw garlic should be eaten every day.

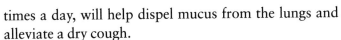

Cuts and wounds

If the cut is deep, it may need to be stitched by a doctor.

Herbal remedies
- To stop bleeding, apply a standard infusion or tincture of yarrow.
- To clean a cut or wound apply a herbal antiseptic which will also aid healing, such as a standard infusion of agrimony, marigold, sage or St John's wort. A gauze square soaked in the infusion and held in place with a light bandage is also effective.
- Apply distilled witch hazel or a thoroughly filtered standard infusion of chickweed or marigold on a pad of cotton wool to the cut to stop the bleeding.
- For minor cuts and wounds, apply a compress made using plantain (plantago lanceolata) leaves. Or if the cut

is fairly deep use a compress of St John's wort.
- After cleansing, apply a little soothing marigold ointment.

Cystitis

This occurs when the bladder becomes inflamed usually through an infection or from a build-up of irritant toxic substances in the urine which are ingested in food. Sexual intercourse can also cause cystitis. It results in burning pain on passing urine, pain in the abdomen and back and the frequent urge to go to the toilet.

Herbal remedies
- Drink plenty of ordinary water or barley water, which has a soothing and mildly diuretic effect, to help flush the germs out of the bladder. To make your own barley water, put 120g of barley in a pan. Pour over enough water to cover it and bring to the boil. Remove from heat, strain and then pour 500ml of cold water over the barley, add the rind of half a lemon and simmer until barley is soft. Leave until lukewarm, then remove barley. Add 20ml–40ml (1–2 tblsp) honey and drink as required.
- A standard infusion of thyme which is anti-inflammatory, or lavender, which is antiseptic, will help ease the condition. Take one teacupful six times a day.

Depression

Long-term depression needs expert help, but in the short-term several herbs have a reputation for lifting the spirits. Herbal remedies can also be used to counter the physical exhaustion which often accompanies this condition.

Herbal remedies
- A standard infusion using any one (or a combination) of the following herbs will help soothe the nerves and brighten the mood. Choose from: lemon balm, St John's wort or vervain.
- Oats are also beneficial to the nervous system. Eat either mixed with a little warm water as porridge or use as a tincture (*see* **blood pressure, low**).
- Try a relaxing herbal bath by adding a standard infusion of lavender to relieve irritability, exhaustion and to lift depression.

Diarrhoea
(see also **colitis**)

This can be caused by poor diet, but usually it is due to an infection or irritation of part of the digestive tract. If symptoms persist for more than 48 hours, consult a doctor.

Herbal remedies
- Drink plenty of water to replace lost fluids.
- A standard infusion made with the astringent herbs agrimony or plantain (plantago major) is beneficial. Pour 500 ml of boiling water over 90g (3 tblsp) fresh or 30g (1 tblsp) dried finely chopped herb. Cover and allow to stand for 15 minutes then strain. Take 60 ml (3 tblsp) three times a day.
- A cup of a standard infusion of chamomile, lady's mantle, meadowsweet or thyme – all mildly antiseptic – taken three times a day will help relieve any pain.
- If the condition is brought on by stress, a standard

infusion of either chamomile, lemon balm or valerian makes a calming relaxant.
- If there is an infection, fast for a day, but don't forget to take in plenty of fluids and then include raw garlic in your diet or take a standard infusion of echinacea, both of which are natural antibiotics.
- Take 10g (1 tsp) of either slippery elm powder dissolved in 150ml (1 cup) of hot water or a standard decoction made with marshmallow root to help settle the digestion and soothe the whole tract.

Dizziness

Most attacks of dizziness are harmless and are the result of a momentary fall in blood pressure or a diminished supply of blood to the brain. If you experience the sensation of unsteadiness and lightheadedness, it is best to sit down and put your head between your knees.

Herbal remedies
- Rub an infused herbal oil made with rosemary onto the temples and inhale from your hands.
- Sip a cup of a standard infusion of peppermint to help revive.

Earache
(see also **catarrh, tonsillitis**)

A pain in the ear is often caused by an infection of the middle ear or inflammation of the outer ear canal, or associated conditions such as thick catarrh or tonsillitis. For recurrent ear infections, or glue ear (an accumulation of fluid in the middle ear cavity) look for underlying causes

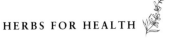

such as chronic throat, tonsil or catarrh problems and avoid dairy products which promote the production of mucus.

Herbal remedies
- Carefully apply 2–3 drops of a herbal infused oil in the ear. Use marshmallow leaves if the problem is in the outer ear. If the condition is accompanied by vertigo and/or nausea, the inner ear could be inflamed and drops of a St John's wort herbal oil should be applied. After applying the drops lie down for a few minutes with the ear that is not affected resting on a pillow.
- Where catarrh of the middle ear is causing problems, drink one cup of a standard infusion of alehoof (ground ivy) three times a day.
- A standard infusion of feverfew, applied as a compress, will help ease discomfort.
- Take raw garlic daily to fight the infection.

Eczema

An inflammation of the skin, usually causing itching. This can be dry and sore or develop blisters that weep and then form dry scales. Eczema can be triggered by stress and poor diet or it can be a hereditary allergic condition, often linked to asthma, psoriasis or hay fever. Foods such as milk products and eggs or substances such as house dust or animal hair can all act as triggers.

Herbal remedies
- A cup of a standard infusion of fresh chickweed taken three times a day, or fresh chickweed juice applied directly to the skin will help relieve the symptoms of itching.

- A standard infusion added to the bath water, using any one (or a combination) of the following herbs will help soothe and heal: agrimony, burdock, chamomile, cleavers, echinacea, fumitory or nettle.
- To nourish the skin, add a handful of fine oatmeal to the bath water, rinsing off with the shower afterwards, and use oatmeal soap.
- To help reduce any inflammation, apply a poultice using either chamomile, echinacea or marigold mixed with a little fine oatmeal.
- To moisturise dry, irritated skin, gently massage in a little chickweed ointment.

Fever
(see also **bronchitis, catarrh, colds, coughs, sore throat**)

A fever, when the body's temperature goes above the normal level of 37°C (98.6°F), is a symptom of the body's fight against infection. It may be accompanied by other symptoms such as shivering, sweating, hot flushes.

Note
A doctor should always be consulted when a child has a fever.

Herbal remedies
- A standard infusion made with elderflowers, peppermint or yarrow will help regulate the temperature. Take 20ml (1 tblsp) every hour.
- To encourage perspiration and eliminate toxins from the body and to fight infection, a standard infusion using any of the following herbs is beneficial: alehoof (ground ivy), catnip, chamomile, elderflowers, feverfew, hyssop, white horehound, lemon balm, lime flowers, peppermint, vervain or yarrow.
- Raw garlic will also help fight infection.

Flatulence
(see also **constipation, diarrhoea, indigestion**)

The most common causes for a build-up of gases in the stomach or bowel are a weak digestion, bad eating habits and stress and anxiety which disturbs the digestion.

Herbal remedies
- Carminative herbs are best for relieving wind and the feeling of bloatedness which often accompanies it. Take as a standard infusion or as a tincture – dilute 10–15 drops in 150ml (1 cup) of water – and drink after a meal. Recommended herbs include: angelica, aniseed, chamomile, fennel and ginger.
- After a meal, sip a cup of a standard infusion of peppermint.

Haemorrhoids

This condition occurs when the veins around the anus or in the rectum become varicose, and therefore swollen, stretched and painful. If bleeding occurs, always consult a doctor. Haemorrhoids or piles are very common during pregnancy and childbirth and often occur during severe cases of constipation, resulting from a diet containing too many highly refined foods and lacking in fibre.

Herbal remedies
- An ointment made with the antiseptic herbs of plantain (plantago major), yarrow or witch hazel leaves, applied to the affected area will help soothe and heal.
- Alternatively, apply a compress using a standard decoction of bistort rhizome or a standard infusion of marigold, nettle or St John's wort.

Hangover

Drink plenty of water before going to bed to prevent dehydration.

Herbal remedies
- A standard infusion of either chamomile, milk thistle, peppermint, thyme or yarrow will help settle the stomach and liver.

Hay fever
(see also **catarrh**)

This inflammation of the mucus membrane of the upper respiratory tract which results in sneezing, running eyes and nose and nasal congestion is an allergic response triggered by various different types of pollen.

Herbal remedies
- Before the hay fever season starts, it's a good idea to boost the immune system. Drink regular standard infusions made with echinacea. Or take a sherry glass of red beetroot juice once a day.
- During the hay fever season, a standard infusion made using either chamomile, echinacea, elderflowers or eyebright (or a combination of any of these herbs) is very effective for reducing discomfort.
- A steam inhalation using chamomile or yarrow flowers will help ease the catarrh and congestion and calm the allergic response.
- Apply soothing cold compresses of distilled witch hazel to the eyelids to ease discomfort.

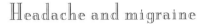

Headache and migraine

A headache or migraine may be a warning sign of stress or fatigue but can also relate to a variety of different conditions such as hormonal imbalances, premenstrual tension, allergies, high blood pressure and poor diet. Migraine sufferers in particular should avoid eating cheese, chocolate, shellfish, orange, bananas and drinking coffee.

Herbal remedies
- Feverfew is the primary herbal remedy for migraine headaches and has been the subject of several clinical studies proving its medicinal benefits. Traditionally, feverfew leaves were eaten fresh between two slices of bread, but a recent study revealed that when taken in this form the herb caused mouth ulcers in 11 per cent of those tested. Therefore taking feverfew in tincture form is now recommended. Make the tincture using fresh leaves, in a strength of one part of leaves to five parts of a 25 per cent alcohol. The recommended dosage is 5 ml (1 tsp) three times a day while symptoms last.
- Alternatively, at the first signs of headache pain, drink one cup of a standard infusion using either chamomile, feverfew, hawthorn, lavender, lemon balm, rosemary or sage.
- A warm herbal bath, adding 4–5 drops of lavender essential oil will help relax muscles and soothe pain.
- For tension and stress-related headaches, a standard infusion of lavender, valerian or vervain will help to calm and relax.
- A standard infusion using a combination of chamomile, hawthorn and peppermint can also help ease a migraine.

Herpes

The outbreak of painful blisters (either as herpes simplex – cold sores and genital herpes – or herpes zoster – shingles) is caused by the activation of the herpes virus that lays dormant in the body. It can be triggered by being run-down, following a poor diet, suffering from an infection or stress, and – in the case of cold sores – when the temperature is raised, such as in a fever or during prolonged exposure to the sun.

Herbal remedies
- To boost the body's resistance take echinacea, either as a standard infusion, or as a tincture – use 5–10 drops diluted in 150 ml (1 cup) of water.
- For shingles, combine echinacea with St John's wort and oats in a standard infusion to support the nervous system.
- For cold sores, dab on a standard infusion or diluted tincture of either myrrh or marigold stems.
- To inhibit the multiplication of cold sores apply either tincture of lemon balm or St John's wort infused oil, made using the flowers, as soon as the sensation of the blisters coming up is felt.
- To help relieve the pain of the blisters of shingles, gently apply with cotton wool a standard infusion made using marigold and St John's wort.

Indigestion
(see also **acid stomach, flatulence**)

This feeling of discomfort in the upper abdomen or chest can be caused through eating too much rich or spicy food, by stress, smoking, or drinking too much alcohol or drinks high in caffeine such as tea or coffee. It can also be triggered by upset or excitement.

Herbal remedies

- At the first sign of discomfort, mix 30g (1 tblsp) of slippery elm powder with a little warm water into a paste. Stir in 150ml (1 cup) of hot water, sweeten with honey if desired, and drink.
- A warm standard infusion made using a combination of the following herbs: fennel, ginger, marshmallow, meadowsweet, milk thistle or peppermint will help calm and settle the stomach.
- If suffering from tension, add either chamomile or lemon balm to your chosen standard infusion.
- To prevent an attack, take a cup of a standard decoction of burdock or dandelion root, or a standard infusion of angelica, milk thistle or white horehound half an hour before a meal.

Insomnia

The inability to sleep can be caused by a wide variety of different factors. Being run-down and overtired, suffering from high levels of tension, anxiety and stress, and/or digestive problems or nutritional deficiencies can all lead to sleepless nights. There are steps you can take to help yourself get a good night's rest. Never eat a large meal just before going to bed and avoid late-night drinks containing caffeine such as tea, coffee or hot chocolate. There are also certain herbs which can be used to great effect to provide a totally natural and non-addictive remedy to help aid restful sleep.

Herbal remedies
- Drinking a cup of a warm standard infusion of either valerian, to reduce tension, or relaxing chamomile or lime flowers will reduce anxiety and promote restful sleep.
- Other herbal sleeping aids including 5ml (1 tsp) of cowslip tincture, made from cowslip flowers, taken last thing at night or by having a warm bath, with a relaxing standard infusion of lavender added to the water, before going to bed.

Irritable Bowel Syndrome
(see also **colitis, constipation, diarrhoea, flatulence**)

In this condition the bowel becomes over-active, often resulting in bouts of both diarrhoea and constipation. Other symptoms include flatulence, back pain, a feeling of bloatedness and general tiredness. The lining of the bowel can react to tension and therefore IBS can be triggered by anxiety, stress and nervous disorders, as well as food intolerance and a poor diet. If there is any sign of bleeding from the bowel, see a doctor immediately.

Herbal remedies
- A standard decoction of marshmallow root which produces a mucilage (gel-like substance) that acts as a protective coating to the bowel will help ease any spasm or pain.
- A hot standard infusion combining chamomile and valerian will help to calm or a standard infusion of agrimony will help to tone and heal.

Laryngitis
(see also **sore throat, tonsillitis**)

This is the inflammation of the larynx (or voice box) which leads to hoarseness or even loss of voice.

Herbal remedies
- A steam inhalation is very soothing. Use chamomile for its anti-inflammatory and antiseptic properties.
- Or try a compress using a standard infusion of either hyssop, sage or thyme applied around the throat and chest for instant relief.
- Gargle with a standard infusion of sage or rosemary or tincture of myrrh – use 20 drops diluted in 150ml (1 cup) of water.
- Drink a cup of a standard infusion made with echinacea and thyme every two hours to help fight the infection.
- Add fennel if you have a tight cough and either elderflowers or yarrow if there is a fever.

Menopause

This is the time when the follicles in a woman's ovaries stop producing eggs and monthly periods cease. It usually takes place between the ages of 45 to 55 and can be accompanied by a number of different symptoms as the balance of hormones in the body changes. These symptoms include hot flushes, night sweats and palpitations, anxiety, insomnia, lack of concentration, mood swings and depression.

Herbal remedies
- Regular drinks of a standard infusion made from either chamomile or valerian will act as a general relaxant.

- If hot flushes are a problem, a standard infusion of lady's mantle, St John's wort or sage will help.
- For palpitations and anxiety, a standard infusion of valerian or lemon balm will calm and relax.

Morning sickness

Sickness during the early stages of pregnancy is extremely common.

Herbal remedies
- Sip an infusion of fresh ginger regularly, or nibble on ginger biscuits or mix a pinch of ginger powder in a little water and sip.
- A cup of a warm standard infusion of chamomile is also effective.

Mouth ulcers

These blisters often occur when the body is run-down or highly stressed. Or they can occur as a result of too much dairy produce in the diet.

Herbal remedies
- Gargle with a mouthwash made from antiseptic herbs such as myrrh diluted as a tincture – use 20 drops diluted in 150 ml (1 cup) of warm water – or a standard infusion of bistort, herb Robert or sage.

Note
While there are some simple herbal remedies which are perfectly safe and very effective, herbs with a strong action must be avoided throughout pregnancy. If you are expecting a baby, do check with the A–Z of Herbs (see pages 97–140) before using any herbal remedy.

Nausea and vomiting

Rejection of the body of food or liquids usually has a simple explanation such as irritation of the stomach by infection or over-indulgence in food or alcohol, or it can be a sign of something more serious. If symptoms persist, consult a doctor.

Herbal remedies
- A standard infusion of either aniseed, chamomile, fennel, ginger, black horehound or peppermint will all help settle the stomach.
- A standard infusion of chamomile or thyme will help fight any infection. And if there is an accompanying fever, include either lime flowers or yarrow in the standard infusion.

Nervous tension

Symptoms of a high stress level can take many forms from muscle tension to headaches, palpitations to sweating. Herbs work to counter undue stress by toning and reviving the nervous system.

Herbal remedies
- A standard infusion of either vervain, oats, chamomile, lavender or lemon balm will help calm, tone and boost a depleted nervous system.
- A standard infusion of chamomile, lemon balm or valerian will help soothe the nerves and relax tense muscles.
- For restlessness, tremors and phobias, take a cup of a standard decoction of valerian root, three times a day.
- Cowslip flowers act as a relaxing sedative for stress-

related tension. Drink one cup of the standard infusion made with the petals, three times a day.
- Take a relaxing herbal bath, adding a standard infusion made with any one (or a combination) of the following herbs: chamomile, cowslip flowers, lavender, lime flowers, thyme, valerian or vervain.

Painful periods

Many women experience cramp-like pains in the lower abdomen at the beginning of their period.

Herbal remedies
- Gently sip a cup of a warm standard infusion of chamomile and valerian, or lady's mantle, three times a day, to ease cramps.

Premenstrual tension

This covers a whole range of symptoms suffered by women – including water retention and bloatedness, food and alcohol cravings, weight gain, skin problems, headaches, irritability and mood swings. These are caused by the hormonal changes which take place just before the onset of menstruation.

Herbal remedies
- Take a cup of a standard infusion of chamomile combined with valerian, two or three times a day during the week before a period is due – its calming and slightly diuretic action will help to reduce any water retention.
- Another recommended diuretic herb is dandelion leaves. Take as a standard infusion.

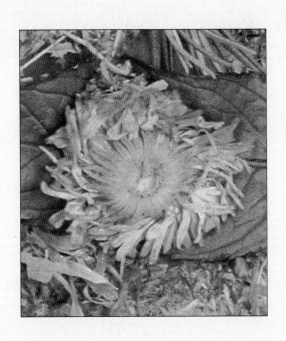

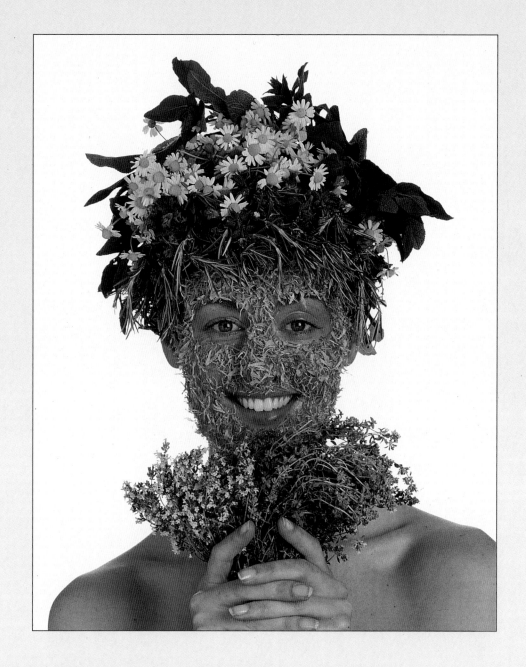

*F*eel beautiful inside and out - and use the unique therapeutic properties of
herbs together with their glorious fragrance to enhance the
appearance and lift the spirit.

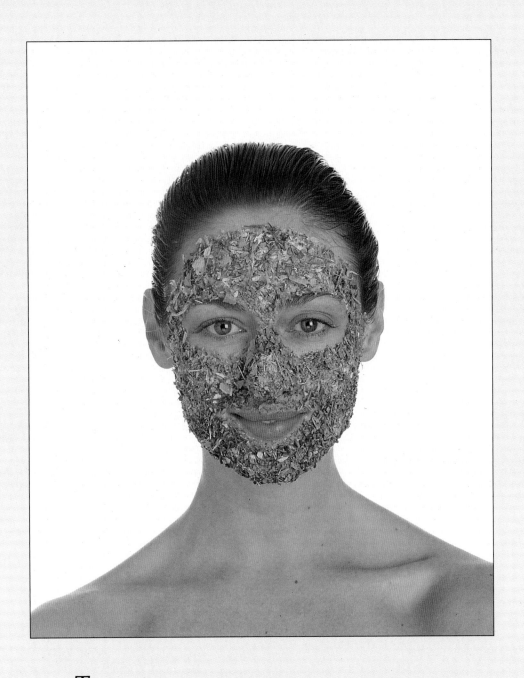

*T*reat yourself to a herbal deep cleansing face pack or mask once a week to remove all traces of stale make-up and help keep the complexion radiant and clear.

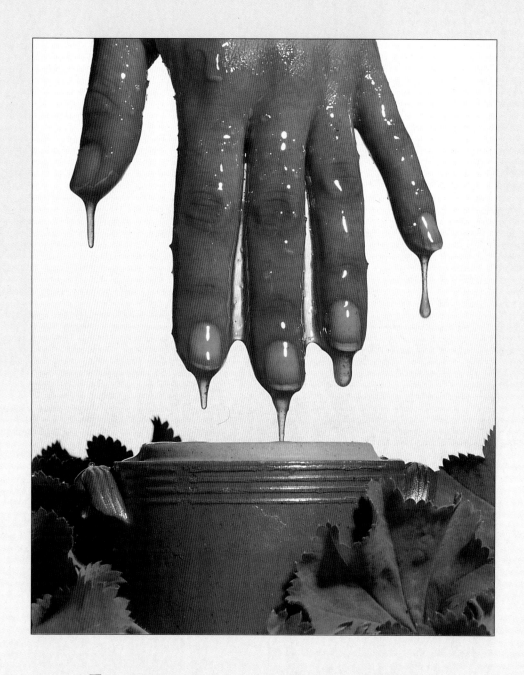

*For a rich moisturising treatment for hands use a conditioner made
with lady's mantle and to strengthen nails, dip them in honey
mixed with a little infusion of horsetail.*

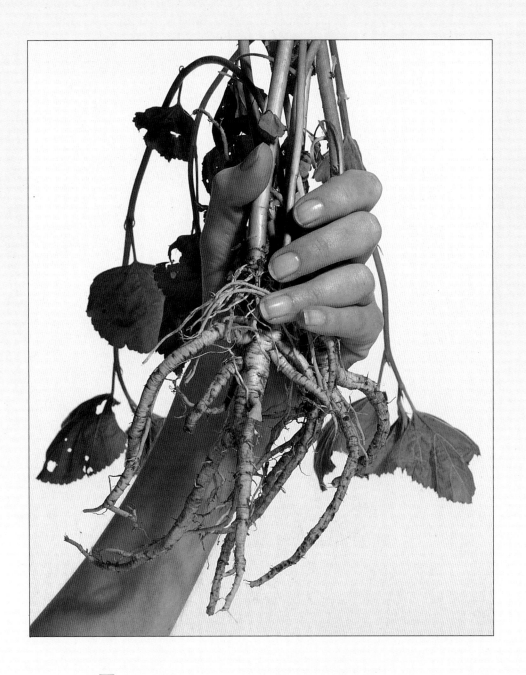

*T*he mucilage obtained from marshmallow root makes a perfect
repair cream for dry, chapped hands.

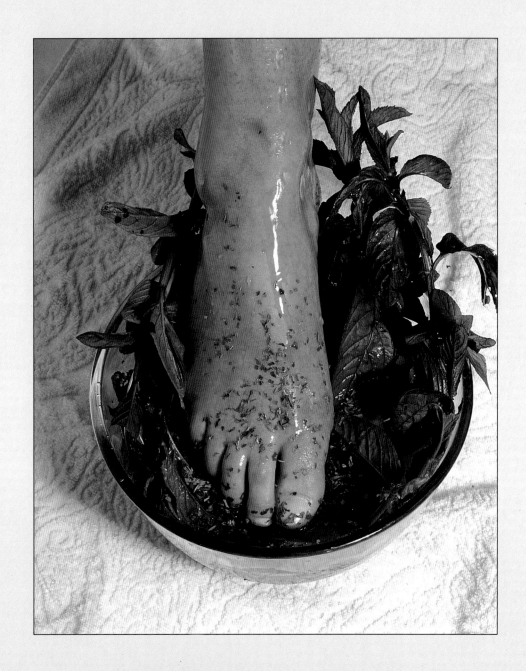

*D*on't neglect your feet. At the end of a tiring day, a
refreshing peppermint footbath works wonders.

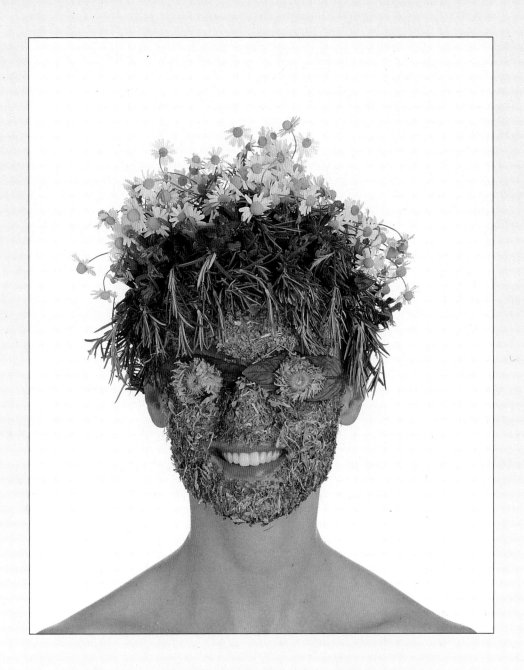

*P*amper yourself with herbs: rosemary and chamomile make fabulous
conditioners for the hair and the soothing and gentle properties
of chickweed, lime flower and marigold are
all kind to the skin.

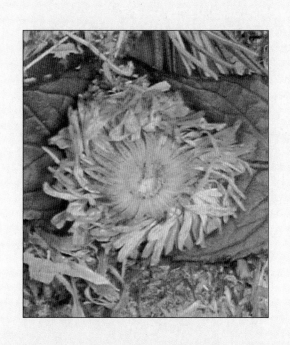

- For headaches, a standard infusion of relaxants such as chamomile or lavender or tincture of feverfew – take 10–20 drops diluted in 150 ml (1 cup) of water – should ease the pain.

Psoriasis

This condition, which results in raised, red scaly patches on the skin, often runs in families and is thought to be caused by some kind of disturbance to the immune system which can be triggered by illness or emotional stress. For any treatment to be successful, all dairy products, red meat, sugar and shellfish should be avoided and carbohydrate intake reduced.

Herbal remedies
- Blood cleansing herbs such as burdock and dandelion root taken as a standard decoction will help the purification and healing process. Do be sure to build up the dose gradually. Start by taking 3 ml (½ tsp) a day, building up to 20 ml (1 tblsp) after a week.
- A standard infusion of either chamomile, valerian or vervain will help to relax the nervous system and/or echinacea, during the inflammatory stage of the condition, can be taken to boost the immune system.
- Externally an ointment made using fresh chickweed or cleavers will help soothe the condition and keep the skin moisturised.
- Or add a standard infusion of either cleavers, marigold, St John's wort or yarrow to a bath.

Rheumatism
(see also **arthritis**)

Rheumatism is a term that covers a number of different conditions which all involve a painful swelling and stiffness to the joints and muscles which in severe cases can sometimes lead to a deformity of the affected area. Following a well-balanced diet that avoids red meat, sugar and high levels of alcohol will help ease the condition. There are also a number of herbal remedies to be recommended.

Herbal remedies
- Dilute 2–3 drops of eucalyptus oil or lavender essential oil in 5 ml (1 tsp) of vegetable oil and massage into the affected area to help reduce inflammation.
- A standard infusion made with anti-inflammatory herbs such as echinacea or meadowsweet will help this condition.
- A standard decoction using burdock root or dandelion root or a standard infusion made with either nettle or parsley will help rid the body of unwanted toxins that build up around the joints and contribute towards the inflammation.
- A standard infusion of valerian will help to ease any pain.

Sciatica

A painful condition affecting the sciatic nerve which results in pain, usually in the buttock or thigh, but can sometimes extend down the leg to the foot, and may be accompanied by numbness. It can be caused by simply putting pressure on the nerve through turning awkwardly or, more commonly, through a slipped disc in the back.

Herbal remedies

- To ease the pain, rub a herbal infused oil made with St John's wort flowers into the affected area.
- Alternatively, apply frequent hot compresses made using a standard infusion of chamomile or valerian.
- Take a standard infusion of either chamomile, lime flowers or valerian to help relax the muscles and lessen the pain.

Sore throat
(see also **laryngitis, tonsillitis**)

A sore throat is often the first symptom of a cold, flu or laryngitis.

Herbal remedies

- As a preventative measure take raw garlic to guard against infection.
- At the first sign of the throat feeling rough or raw, gargle with a standard infusion using a strong herbal antibiotic such as echinacea, myrrh, sage or thyme.
- A warm cup of a standard infusion made with any one (or a combination) of the following antiseptic herbs: elderflowers, eyebright and hyssop with 20 ml (1 tblsp) of honey added will soothe and heal.
- Add peppermint to the infusion in cases of fever or flu, or alehoof (ground ivy) if accompanied by catarrh.
- If the neck glands are swollen, gargle with a cup of a standard infusion of marigold to help reduce swelling and ease tenderness.

Sprains

These occur when the ligaments that support the joints are overstretched or torn.

Herbal remedies
- To ease the swelling, apply a cool compress made with a standard infusion of marigold or witch hazel leaves, or a standard decoction of witch hazel bark.
- Or fill an ice cube tray with the above strained infusion or decoction and freeze, then apply these herbal cubes to the affected area.
- A poultice using St John's wort or marigold, held with a firm bandage over the sprain, will ease pain and inflammation.

Sunburn

Over-exposure to the sun's rays can result in serious burns and sunstroke. Always make sure that the body is thoroughly protected at all times.

Herbal remedies
- For immediate relief, cover affected area with live natural yogurt or buttermilk.
- Add a standard infusion of chamomile to a lukewarm bath to relieve sunburnt skin.

Thrush

This fungal infection, also known as candidiasis, flourishes when the immune system is weakened by infection, long-term or repeated use of antibiotics or nutritional deficiencies, especially iron or zinc.

Herbal remedies
- Antifungal herbs include chamomile, marigold or thyme – take as standard infusions or tinctures. Add echinacea to boost the immune system.
- A standard infusion using any one (or a combination) of the above herbs added to your bath will help ease vaginal thrush.
- For oral thrush use any one (or a combination) of the above recommended herbs in a standard infusion and use as a mouthwash.
- Eat raw garlic to help fight the infection.

Tonsillitis
(see also **sore throat**)

This inflammation of the tonsils due to an infection produces swollen glands in the neck, a very sore throat and sometimes a fever. It is highly infectious and is most common in children. If symptoms persist more than 24 hours, consult a doctor.

Herbal remedies
- To fight the infection, gargle using a standard infusion of any one (or a combination) of the following antiseptic herbs: alehoof (ground ivy), chamomile, sage or thyme, adding hot lemon and honey.
- Alternatively, add 20 drops of tincture of myrrh to 150ml (1 cup) of warm water and use as a mouthwash.
- Alternatively, more soothing is to drink a cup of a hot standard infusion made using chamomile, echinacea or marigold, adding lemon and honey.
- Apply compresses of any of the above infusions to the throat and neck to ease soreness.
- Take raw garlic to clear the infection.

Toothache

If pain persists, consult your dentist.

Herbal remedies
- To ease pain apply oil of cloves, which has antiseptic properties, on a cotton bud to the affected area.
- If the pain is really bad, sip a cup of a standard infusion of valerian.
- If a tooth has just been taken out, make up a mouthwash and gargle frequently with a standard infusion of marigold or 20 drops of tincture of myrrh diluted in 150ml (1 cup) of water.

Travel sickness
(see also **nausea and vomiting**)

Herbal remedies
- The volatile oil found in ginger provides the best remedy. Either chew the fresh root or crystallised stem ginger, or sip on ginger beer or a pinch of ginger powder dissolved in a little water.
- A standard infusion of black horehound or peppermint will also help settle the stomach.

Varicose veins

Veins, most commonly in the legs, become enlarged or twisted, due to defective valves. The affected area often aches severely and can cause swelling of the feet and ankles. The disorder tends to run in families and is worsened by prolonged standing, a lack of exercise or when pregnant or overweight.

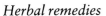

Herbal remedies

- For immediate relief, sit down with the legs raised above hip level.
- Hose the veins with a strong jet of cold water for 4–5 minutes every morning.
- Tone the affected veins by bathing them with a standard infusion of either marigold flowers or witch hazel leaves.

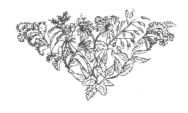

5

The A–Z of herbs

In this chapter you'll find a comprehensive index in alphabetical order of over 50 of the most widely used and easily available herbs. Each entry gives a brief background to the plant, the parts used, any cautions which should be noted and the relevant medicinal and beauty uses of the herb which can be found in Chapters 3 and 4, The beauty of herbs (page 21) and Herbs for health (page 55).

Agrimony
Agrimonia eupatoria

It takes its name from the Greek word *argemone*, meaning 'cataract', because it was considered to have special properties to help heal eye complaints. The Anglo Saxons used it to treat warts and snakebites and believed it would protect against goblins and evil. Monks grew agrimony in their medicine gardens as a cure for stomach ache and to treat open wounds. In the 1800s it was valued as a substitute for the still expensive tea, or as an addition to make tea go further and to add a delicate aroma.

DESCRIPTION A lightly scented perennial with hairy, divided leaves at ground level. It is also

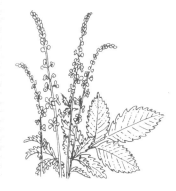

sometimes known as 'church steeples' due to its tall, tapering spikes of bright yellow flowers that appear in the summer.

PARTS USED   Stem, leaves.

HEALTH   As a mild astringent, it is an effective herb to tone the stomach. Use for athlete's foot, colitis, conjunctivitis, cuts and wounds, diarrhoea, eczema, irritable bowel syndrome.

Angelica
Angelica archangelica

This herb was dedicated to heathen gods and featured in pagan festivals. It is said to have got its name because the medicinal qualities of the plant were revealed to a monk by an angel who told him it was a cure for the plague. From then on it was considered to protect against evil and infectious disease. Culpeper recommended it for conditions ranging from dog bites to gout. Today the crystallised stalks of angelica are used in decorative confectionery and in the making of liqueurs such as Chartreuse and Benedictine.

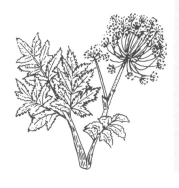

DESCRIPTION   A biennial with a thick, fleshy root, hollow stems, toothed leaves and clusters of greenish-white flowers in early summer.

PARTS USED   Roots, seeds, fresh leaves.

CAUTION   Avoid large or regular doses in pregnancy as it can act as a uterine stimulant.

HEALTH   A stimulating, warming, antiseptic herb recommended for acid stomach, bronchitis, colds, coughs, flatulence, indigestion.

BEAUTY   *Body:* bath infusion to relieve tired/aching muscles. *Feet:* deodorising footbath.

Anise/aniseed
Pimpinella anisum

One of the most ancient herbs, aniseed was cultivated by the Egyptians in quantity and later by the Greeks and Arabs, to supply food, drink and medicine from its leaves and seeds. At Roman weddings, a cake flavoured with aniseed was part of the marriage feast because it was considered to have great aphrodisiac qualities. In the Middle Ages too, as well as being used as a spice and a carminative medicine, it also became known as a principal ingredient of aphrodisiac potions.

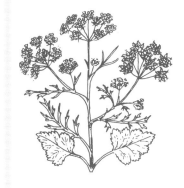

DESCRIPTION	An aromatic annual with a thin root and round, lobed mid-green lower leaves and finely divided, feathery upper leaves. Small, whitish flowers late summer to early autumn followed by brownish, ribbed, oval fruit.
PARTS USED	Seeds.
HEALTH	A soothing, decongestant, pungent herb, recommended for bad breath, colds, flatulence, nausea and vomiting.
BEAUTY	*Mouth:* breath freshener. *Body:* herbal all-over body tonic.

Basil
Ocimum basilicum

The name of this herb comes from the Greek word *basileus*, meaning 'king', indicating the esteem with which this herb was regarded. A native of India, it is deemed a sacred plant by the Hindus and is grown outside temples. The plant is also often kept inside the house, not just because it is deemed holy but because it is an effective insect repellent. In Egypt it is scattered over graves. Basil has been growing in Britain since the sixteenth century when it was believed that it could only be cultivated by a beautiful woman. It was given and received as a token of love.

DESCRIPTION	A highly aromatic annual with smooth, slightly curved green or red leaves and small white flowers in the summer, followed by small, black seeds.
PARTS USED	Whole herb.
HEALTH	A calming, mildly antiseptic herb recommended for bites and stings.
BEAUTY	*Body:* relaxing bath infusion.

Bistort
Polygonum bistorta

The name bistort means twice twisted and refers to the underground stem of this herb which is bent like the letter 'S'. Old herbalists called it snakeweed, and it was not introduced for use in herbal medicine in this country until the Renaissance.

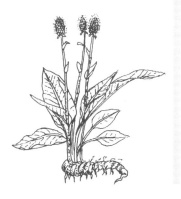

DESCRIPTION	A hardy perennial with broad, oval leaves and knobbly twisted roots. It produces spikes of pink flowers in late spring.
PARTS USED	Rhizome (where the stem meets the root).
HEALTH	The rhizome of this herb is a powerful astringent and anti-inflammatory recommended for haemorrhoids and mouth ulcers.

Burdock
Arctium lappa

Burdock is an ancient and versatile herb best known as a blood purifier in the tonic dandelion and burdock wine. According to folklore, burdock seeds hung in a bag around the neck were believed to protect against rheumatism. Its roots are eaten by the Japanese as a vegetable for the dietary fibre they contain.

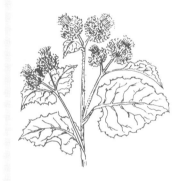

DESCRIPTION	A biennial with a large taproot, big arrow-shaped leaves and thistle-like purple flowers covered with tiny hooks or burrs.
PARTS USED	Root, leaves.
HEALTH	A herbal antibiotic and detoxifying herb. Recommended for acne and spots, arthritis, athlete's foot, boils and sores, bruises, conjunctivitis, eczema, indigestion, psoriasis, rheumatism.
BEAUTY	*Face:* blackheads/problem skin facial steam. *Hair:* recommended for dry/sensitive hair; anti-dandruff; herbal tonic finishing rinse; herbal warm oil repair treatment.

Catnip/catmint
Nepeta cataria

Catmint was said to bring warmth and comfort to 'cold aches and cramps'. Culpeper said that catmint, 'taketh away barrenness . . . and the pains of the mother' and it was used in baths for women 'to make them fruitful'. It has a mint-like smell liked by cats.

DESCRIPTION	A member of the mint family, it has a hairy, four-sided stem, whitish-green pointed

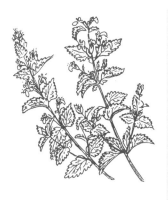

leaves and white to pale-blue, dotted with crimson, flowers.

PARTS USED   The whole herb, ideally just before flowering.

HEALTH   It has a diaphoretic action (promotes sweating) and is recommended for colds and fever.

BEAUTY   *Hair:* recommended for normal hair; improved growth; herbal tonic finishing rinse. *Body:* relaxing bath infusion.

Chamomile

There are two main varieties of chamomile:

Chamomile, German
Chamomilla recutita

The name is derived from the Greek *chamoemelon* meaning 'earth apple' because it was thought that the herb smelled like apples. This plant along with its very close relative, Roman chamomile (see the page opposite), has been used for centuries by herbal practitioners. Chamomile was recommended as far back as 900 BC by Asclepiades, a physician skilled in the use of herbs. It has been called the plants' physician because sickly garden plants have been known to recover when it is planted next to them. The Egyptians dedicated it to the sun and worshipped it above all other herbs for its healing properties. Lawns of it were planted before grass lawns were introduced into our gardens. It is said that Sir Francis Drake played his historic game of bowls on a lawn of clipped chamomile.

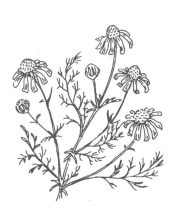

DESCRIPTION   A low-growing aromatic annual with finely divided leaves and daisy-like flowers.

PARTS USED   Flowers.

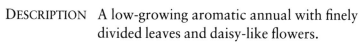

Chamomile, Roman
Chamaemelum nobile

This is a double variety and is best known for lawns as it is more compact in growth. The name *nobile* indicates how highly thought of the plant was by herbalists.

DESCRIPTION	Very similar in appearance to German chamomile, to which it is closely related. It has an almost identical smell and taste. It is perennial rather than annual.
PARTS USED	Flowers.
HEALTH	The relaxant, digestive and anti-inflammatory properties of chamomile make it an invaluable remedy. While German chamomile is preferable, both varieties can be recommended for acid stomach, acne and spots, baldness, burns, catarrh, colds, colitis, conjunctivitis, constipation, diarrhoea, eczema, fever, flatulence, hangover, hay fever, headache and migraine, indigestion, insomnia, irritable bowel syndrome, laryngitis, menopause, morning sickness, nausea and vomiting, nervous tension, painful periods, premenstrual tension, psoriasis, sciatica, sunburn, thrush, tonsillitis.
BEAUTY	*Face:* recommended for oily skin; deep cleansing; blackheads/problem skin facial steam; lavender anti-blemish night cream. *Eyes:* compress to soothe tired, sore and inflamed eyes. *Hair:* recommended for dry/sensitive hair; colour enhancer for blonde/fair; blonde highlighter paste. *Body:* relaxing bath infusion; skin softening milk bath. *Hands:* herbal hand softening infusion. *Feet:* soothing footbath.

Chickweed
Stellaria media

This herb has been used as bird and animal feed since ancient times, as it is one of the few sources of fresh seed during the winter. It was traditionally eaten as a vegetable by poor country folk and was also used to heal wounds and boils.

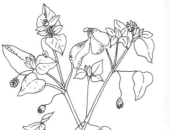

DESCRIPTION	This creeping annual grows in abundance all over Britain. It is a low-growing plant with small, bright green leaves and small, star-like white flowers.
PARTS USED	Whole herb.
HEALTH	The cooling action of this herb makes it valuable for treating irritated skin. Recommended for conjunctivitis, cuts and wounds, eczema, psoriasis.
BEAUTY	*Face:* recommended for oily skin.

Cleavers/Clivers
Galium aparine

The Greeks called this herb *philanthropon*, meaning 'love man', because they believed its clinging habit showed a love of humanity. Today this prolific weed is commonly known as goosegrass. It has been widely used in folk medicine for centuries, and is considered very beneficial in the treatment of skin conditions.

DESCRIPTION	A perennial clinging, creeping herb, its leaves and stalks are covered with hooked bristles with which it grows up shrubs and hedges and spreads over other plants. Tiny,

star-shaped, white flowers appear in June and July.

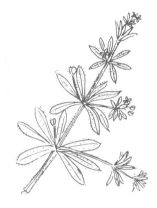

PARTS USED   Whole herb just before flowering.

HEALTH   Reputed for its blood cleansing properties. Recommended for acne and spots, conjunctivitis, eczema, psoriasis.

BEAUTY   *Hair:* recommended for anti-dandruff; added shine and lustre; herbal tonic finishing rinse.

Cowslip
Primula veris

Believed to be the favourite flower of the nightingale who, it was said, only appeared where cowslips flourished. The herb's yellow flowers were believed to symbolise the golden keys that would open the gates of heaven, and as a result the cowslip was also called Peterkeys or Peterwort and dedicated to St Peter. The old herbalists had great faith in its curative properties in cases of palsy and paralytic ailments.

DESCRIPTION   A perennial with green rosettes of wrinkled leaves and a slender stalk crowned by honey-scented yellow flowers in May and June that look like gold chandeliers.

PARTS USED   Root, flowers.

CAUTION   Avoid during pregnancy as this herb can act as a uterine stimulant. Avoid if sensitive to aspirin.

HEALTH   The root is a soothing expectorant recommended for catarrh and coughs. The flowers are good for insomnia and nervous tension.

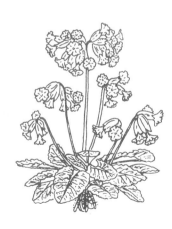

BEAUTY   *Face:* anti-wrinkle lotion. *Body:* relaxing
           bath infusion.

Dandelion
Taraxacum officinale

This herb is also known as *dens leonis* ('lion's teeth')
because of its tooth-shaped leaves. Dandelion was used by
the Arabs in the eleventh century and by the 1500s it was
well established as an official drug of the apothecaries. Its
reputation as a medicine grew as it became a popular salad
herb and coffee substitute.

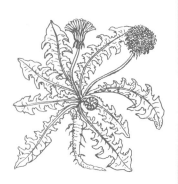

DESCRIPTION Deep root with rosette or spear-shaped,
             serrated leaves and yellow, daisy-like
             flowers.
PARTS USED   Root, leaves.
HEALTH   The leaves are a strong diuretic and blood
             purifier, while the root is a very good tonic.
             Recommended for arthritis, athlete's foot,
             constipation, high blood pressure, indiges-
             tion, premenstrual tension, psoriasis, rheu-
             matism.
BEAUTY   *Face:* recommended for mature/sallow skin;
             deep cleansing facial steam; anti-freckle oil.

Echinacea
Echinacea angustifolia

For over 100 years echinacea or purple coneflower has been
known to increase resistance to infections. Both the North
American Indians and the early settlers used it against
infectious diseases, to clean and heal wounds, and to treat

snakebites. Scientific research has now confirmed its stim-
ulatory effects on the white blood cells that fight infection
and it is being studied as a possible treatment for AIDS.

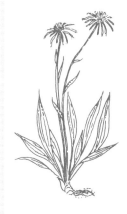

DESCRIPTION   A perennial herb with coarse, hairy stems
and leaves. The purple flowers, which
appear in late summer, are raised daisy-like
cones surrounded with a ring of purple
florets.

PARTS USED   Root.

HEALTH   An excellent herbal antibiotic and blood
purifier which fights infection and boosts
the immune system. Recommended for
acne and spots, athlete's foot, bites and
stings, boils and sores, bronchitis, catarrh,
conjunctivitis, diarrhoea, eczema, hay
fever, herpes, laryngitis, psoriasis, rheumatism, sore throat, thrush, tonsillitis.

Elder
Sambucus nigra

The elder has been held in high esteem throughout the ages
for its considerable medicinal properties. With its Biblical
associations – it is referred to as the wood from which the
crucifixion cross was made and was said to be the type of
tree from which Judas hanged himself – elder is a symbol
of sorrow and death. But it also has associations with
magic. It is considered lucky to plant elder but unlucky to
dig it up. Sprigs hung in the house were said to keep away
evil witches. Its medicinal uses are so varied it's been
christened 'the peoples' medicine chest'.

DESCRIPTION   A shrub or small tree with broad, dentated

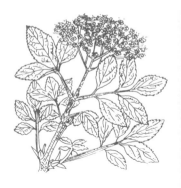

leaves and clusters of small, cream, strongly perfumed flowers in the spring which are followed by purple-black berries.

PARTS USED Flowers, leaves, berries, bark.

CAUTION Elderberries should never be eaten uncooked nor should the raw juice be taken, as both can cause diarrhoea. Also avoid using the bark during pregnancy.

HEALTH An excellent all-round herbal remedy with expectorant, anti-catarrhal, anti-inflammatory, diuretic and astringent properties. Recommended for bronchitis, colds, conjunctivitis, coughs, fever, hay fever, laryngitis, sore throat.

BEAUTY *Face:* recommended for dry/sensitive skin; mature/sallow skin; mature/sallow skin facial steam; elderflower and honey facial scrub; elderflower toner for thread veins. *Eyes:* compress to reduce puffiness and add sparkle. *Hair:* recommended for oily hair; anti-dandruff; colour enhancer for grey and dark hair. *Body:* reviving bath infusion; skin softening milk bath. *Feet:* soothing footbath.

Elecampane
Inula helenium

This herb is said to be named after Helen of Troy, who was supposedly gathering elecampane when she was abducted by Paris. Elecampane was well known to the ancient Greeks and Romans, who used it as a digestive tonic after too much feasting and over-indulging. Its root contains inulin, which was used in the making of throat lozenges and, throughout the ages, elecampane was used to treat many illnesses from whooping cough to kidney troubles.

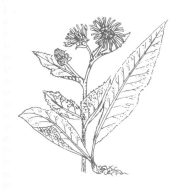

DESCRIPTION	A perennial with a deep taproot, which when dried smells of violets and has a sharp, bitter flavour. It has stout, hairy stems branched at the top and long, pointed, coarsely toothed green leaves with a downy-grey underside and large, yellow flowers like small sunflowers.
PARTS USED	Root.
HEALTH	An expectorant herb recommended for asthma, bronchitis, catarrh, coughs.
BEAUTY	*Face:* blackheads/problem skin facial steam.

Eyebright
Euphrasia officinalis

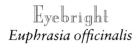

Eyebright was named after one of the three Greek Graces. First records of its medicinal use are from the fourteenth century when it was recommended to 'strengthen the head, eyes and memory'. The sixteenth-century herbalist William Coles said its combination of colours gave it the appearance of a blood-shot eye and so indicated its use as a cure for eye diseases. It therefore became known by apothecaries as Ocularis and Opthalmica.

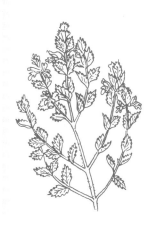

DESCRIPTION	An annual with square, leafy stems, oval, toothed leaves, and two-lipped red or purple flowers, spotted with yellow.
PARTS USED	Whole herb.
HEALTH	An antiseptic, anti-inflammatory, anti-catarrhal remedy, recommended for

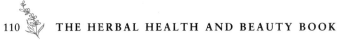

catarrh, colds, conjunctivitis, hay fever, sore throat.

BEAUTY   *Eyes:* compress to soothe tired, sore and inflamed eyes; compress to reduce puffiness and add sparkle; eye gel.

Fennel

Foeniculum vulgare

Fennel is one of the oldest cultivated plants and was much valued by the Romans who called it *foeniculum*, 'little hay', because of its fine, hair-like leaves. Roman warriors took fennel to keep in good health while Roman women ate it as a slimming aid. With its healing properties also recognized, in 812AD the Holy Roman Emperor Charlemagne declared that fennel was essential in every imperial garden. In medieval times it was thought to have magical powers and was hung over doors to protect against witches.

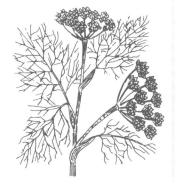

DESCRIPTION   Hardy perennial with a ribbed stem, feathery, aromatic leaves and yellow flowers followed by fruit that taste of anise.

PARTS USED   Seeds.

CAUTION   Best avoided during pregnancy as it can act as a uterine stimulant.

HEALTH   A calming herb with a gentle expectorant action. Recommended for asthma, catarrh, flatulence, indigestion, laryngitis, nausea and vomiting.

BEAUTY   *Face:* recommended for normal skin; deep cleansing facial steam. *Eyes:* compress to reduce puffiness and add sparkle. *Hair:* recommended for normal hair; herbal tonic finishing rinse. *Hands:* herbal hand softening infusion. *Body:* reviving bath infusion; bath infusion to relieve tired and aching muscles.

Feverfew
Tanacetum parthenium

Folk medicine used this herb for many conditions, including nervous complaints, a treatment for arthritis and a general tonic. But it is called feverfew from its older Latin name, *febrifugia*, meaning 'to drive away fevers'. Culpeper wrote that feverfew in wine might help those 'troubled with melancholy and heaviness or sadness of spirits'. Today, feverfew has been the subject of scientific trials proving its effectiveness in treating migraine.

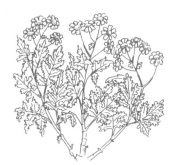

DESCRIPTION A perennial with yellowy-green, pointed leaves with flat, daisy-like flowers in summer.

PARTS USED Whole herb.

CAUTION Feverfew should be avoided in pregnancy. Chewing fresh leaves can trigger an allergic response in the form of mouth ulcers in some cases.

HEALTH An anti-inflammatory, and generally recommended for earache, fever, headache and migraine, premenstrual tension.

Fumitory
Fumaria officinalis

Both its common and botanical names derive from the Latin word for smoke because from a distance, and growing in mass, fumitory gives the appearance of smoke swirling off the ground. It was believed that the smoke it gave off when burned repelled evil spirits. Since Roman times physicians have valued fumitory for its purifying properties and it has been used as a general tonic and a treatment for liver complaints.

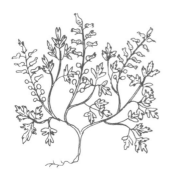

DESCRIPTION	A climbing annual plant with silvery-grey, segmented leaves and the small, pinkish-white flowers with purple tips grow in spikes.
PARTS USED	Whole herb.
HEALTH	As a blood cleanser this herb helps to correct a sluggish digestion. Recommended for constipation and eczema.
BEAUTY	*Face:* recommended for normal skin.

Garlic
Allium sativum

Garlic was first known to the Chinese in 2000 BC and has been used medicinally by them ever since. Divine honours were paid to this strong-smelling herb. The Egyptian pharaohs are said to have placed garlic in their tombs and also to have fed it to their slaves for strength. It was one of the staple foods of Egypt where it grew in abundance. It was believed to have magical powers and was carried as a talisman in China, Japan, Greece and Turkey. German miners took it with them into the mines to ward off evil spirits and in country districts it was put in the stockings of children who had whooping cough. Today it is being closely investigated for its effect on reducing cholesterol and lowering blood pressure and also for its anti-cancer properties.

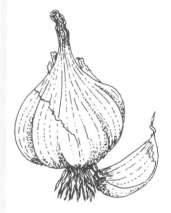

DESCRIPTION	Thin and flat leaves and a spherical flower-head of tiny greenish-white or pink flowers appears in midsummer. The bulb is covered in white papery skin and has 8–15 cloves. The plant has no smell until crushed or broken which is when its characteristic odour is released.
PARTS USED	Cloves.
CAUTION	Garlic can irritate the stomach. Due to its distinct pungent flavour, it can also cause breath odour.
HEALTH	A very good herbal antibiotic which fights infection and has been found to lower high blood pressure and help reduce the level of cholesterol in the blood. Recommended for boils and sores, bronchitis, colds, coughs, diarrhoea, earache, fever, high blood pressure, sore throat, thrush, tonsillitis.

Ginger
Zingiber officinalis

Originally from Asia, ginger has been one of the most important trade items of the Far East since antiquity. While the Romans valued ginger as an Oriental spice and added it to many of their favourite culinary dishes, Hippocrates and the ancient Greeks used ginger as a medicine. It wasn't introduced into England until around 1600.

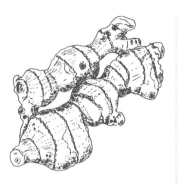

DESCRIPTION A perennial with a thick, tuberous root, long, tapering leaves and purple flowers. The roots are harvested after the leaves die in the autumn.

PARTS USED Root.

HEALTH A very good circulatory stimulant which also strengthens the lungs and is carminative to the digestive tract. Recommended for bad breath, colds, constipation, flatulence, indigestion, low blood pressure, morning sickness, nausea and vomiting, travel sickness.

Hawthorn
Crataegus oxycantha

Hawthorn has a long history of legend attached to it, the most famous being that it was reputedly used for Christ's crown of thorns. In ancient times hawthorn was taken for gout, fever, pleurisy and insomnia. Nowadays it is considered one of the most useful remedies for conditions affecting the heart and circulation.

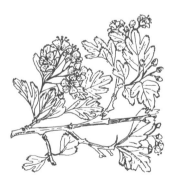

DESCRIPTION This deciduous shrub or small bush has lobed, dark-green leaves with white flowers in the summer and oval, red berries in the autumn.

PARTS USED Flowers, leaves, fruit.

HEALTH A herbal remedy known for its benefits to the heart and circulation. Recommended for arthritis, headache and migraine, high blood pressure.

Herb Robert
Geranium robertianum

An old medicinal plant which was ascribed to St Robert in the Middle Ages. The herb also gets its name from the Greek *gheranos*, 'a crane', because of the resemblance of the fruit to the beak of this bird. According to the seventeenth-century Doctrine of Signatures, its red colour symbolised its therapeutic qualities. It was considered good for regenerating the blood and was prescribed for internal haemorrhages and diabetes.

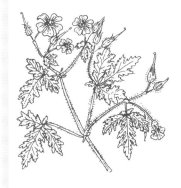

DESCRIPTION	This annual or biennial plant has a red stem with hairy leaves, a small taproot and pinkish-red flowers. It also has an unpleasant smell.
PARTS USED	Leaves, flowers.
HEALTH	An astringent herb. Recommended for acne and spots, bruises, conjunctivitis, mouth ulcers.
BEAUTY	*Face:* oily skin facial steam.

Horehound, black
Ballota nigra

A poor relation of white horehound, this herb has a very strong unpleasant smell. Black horehound's botanical name comes from the Greek word, *ballo*, 'to reject'. However, Culpeper recommended it to be eaten with salt to 'cure the bites of mad dogs'.

DESCRIPTION	A hairy perennial with an unpleasant smell with a short, stout woody root and branched stems. The dull green egg-shaped

leaves are arranged in pairs on the stem and covered in soft, grey hairs. Dull purple flowers from June to October.

PARTS USED Leaves, flowers.

HEALTH A gentle herbal relaxant that helps to counteract sickness. Recommended for nausea and vomiting, travel sickness.

Horehound, white
Marrubium vulgare

One of the oldest and most reliable cough remedies known, white horehound was used by the Egyptian pharaohs to treat many other ailments too. It was also held to be an antidote to various poisons.

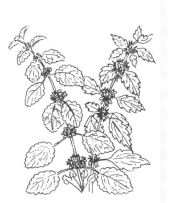

DESCRIPTION A perennial with hairy, square stems and oval, wrinkled leaves. Small, white flowers bloom in summer. It has a sharp, bitter taste but a sweet-smelling scent.

PARTS USED Whole herb, collected during flowering.

CAUTION All infusions should always be freshly made each time. Its bitter taste may be sweetened by adding 5 ml (1 tsp) of honey.

HEALTH This herb has an excellent expectorant action, recommended for asthma, bronchitis, catarrh, colds, coughs, fever, indigestion.

Horsetail
Equisetum arvense

This herb was used since Roman times as a vegetable, animal feed and as a medicine. Culpeper said it was 'very powerful to stop bleeding either inward or outward and eases the swelling, heat and inflammation of the fundamental or privy parts in men and women'. Its fresh plant stems are rich in silica.

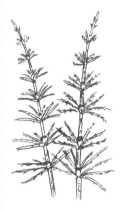

DESCRIPTION	Very fine in appearance, the plant has two types of stem, fertile stems in early spring followed by vegetative stems.
PARTS USED	Vegetative stems.
HEALTH	An astringent herb recommended for conjunctivitis.
BEAUTY	*Face:* recommended for oily skin; oily skin facial steam. *Eyes:* compress to soothe tired, sore and inflamed eyes. *Hair:* recommended for normal hair; anti-dandruff; added shine and lustre; herbal tonic finishing rinse. *Body:* bath infusion to relieve tired/aching muscles. *Hands:* nail strengthener. *Feet:* soothing footbath.

Hyssop
Hyssopus officinalis

Hyssop is mentioned in the Bible as a cleansing plant and it has been used in Mediterranean countries since pre-Christian times for medicinal and culinary purposes. An ancient insecticide, hyssop was put on floors and shelves to repel insects and has been used to treat head lice and internal worms as well as for its more traditional role of easing colds and coughs and aiding digestion.

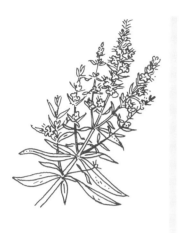

DESCRIPTION	A partially evergreen perennial with thin pointed leaves and small blue, purplish-white, pink or white flowers.
PARTS USED	Whole herb.
CAUTION	Avoid during pregnancy.
HEALTH	As an expectorant and astringent herb, recommended for bronchitis, catarrh, coughs, fever, laryngitis, sore throat.
BEAUTY	*Body:* reviving bath infusion.

Ivy

There are two main varieties of ivy:

Ground ivy (Alehoof)
Glechoma hederacea

This herb was used as a popular folk remedy from the earliest times and was recommended by the Greek physician Galen for its astringent properties in the second century AD. Its name comes from an old English word for the herb, *hofe*.

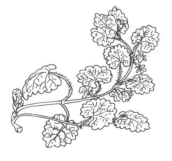

DESCRIPTION	An evergreen, low-growing, perennial it has square stems, dark green, heart-shaped leaves and purple-blue, long spikes of flowers.
PARTS USED	Whole herb.
HEALTH	An anti-catarrhal and healing astringent recommended for catarrh, earache, fever, sore throat, tonsillitis.
BEAUTY	*Body:* reviving bath infusion.

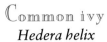

Common ivy
Hedera helix

In ancient times common ivy was thought to be the enemy of the vine and able to prevent drunkenness which is why Bacchus, god of wine, is always shown wearing an ivy wreath. Ivy was also thought to be a symbol of fidelity and Greek priests presented a wreath made of the herb to newly-weds.

DESCRIPTION | A woody, evergreen perennial climbing plant with lobed, triangular leaves.
PARTS USED | Leaves.
CAUTION | The whole plant is poisonous and should only be used externally.
BEAUTY | *Body:* ivy anti-cellulite cream.

Lady's mantle
Alchemilla vulgaris

Its Latin name comes from the fact that this herb was highly regarded by the alchemists of the Middle Ages, who believed the plant had many powers and used it in their search for greater wisdom. The lobed leaves are considered to resemble the scalloped edge of a mantle. Its astringent action meant it was widely used to treat the wounds of soldiers injured on the battlefields in the fifteenth and sixteenth centuries.

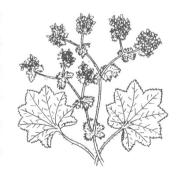

DESCRIPTION | A perennial downy plant with lobed kidney-shaped leaves. Early to midsummer, tiny yellow-green flowers.
PARTS USED | Leaves, flowering tops.
HEALTH | An anti-inflammatory and astringent herb recommended for diarrhoea, menopause, painful periods.

BEAUTY *Face:* recommended for normal skin; deep cleansing mask for normal skin; dry/sensitive skin facial steam. *Body:* bath infusion to relieve tired/aching muscles. *Hands:* herbal hand softening infusion; hand conditioner.

Lavender
Lavandula officinalis

Renowned since Roman times for its wonderful scent and as a flavouring for foods and medicine, lavender gets its name from the Latin *lavare*, 'to wash'. It was the favourite bath water additive of the Greeks and Romans.

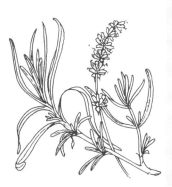

DESCRIPTION Woody, perennial shrub with narrow leaves and blue-violet flowers.

PARTS USED Flowers.

HEALTH A herbal antiseptic. Recommended for acne and spots, bites and stings, cystitis, depression, headache and migraine, high blood pressure, insomnia, nervous tension, premenstrual tension, rheumatism.

BEAUTY *Face:* recommended for mature/sallow skin; facial steam; lavender anti-blemish night cream. *Hair:* recommended for oily hair; anti-dandruff; herbal tonic finishing rinse. *Body:* relaxing bath infusion. *Feet:* refreshing footbath; foot oil.

Lemon balm
Melissa officinalis

Lemon balm gets its name from the Greek *melissa*, meaning 'a honeybee', because bees are very attracted to the herb's flowers, from which they produce extremely good honey. The Romans introduced lemon balm to Britain and it became an important plant in the monastic apothecary garden.

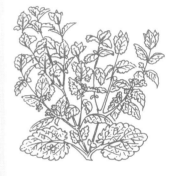

DESCRIPTION	A sweet-scented perennial herb with branched, downy stems and oval to heart-shaped leaves that give off a strong, lemony smell when bruised. The small white or yellowish or pinkish flowers bloom from June to October.
PARTS USED	Leaves.
HEALTH	This fragrant herb is a good sedative for the heart and circulation, aids digestion and relaxes tension. Recommended for depression, diarrhoea, fever, headache and migraine, herpes, high blood pressure, indigestion, menopause, nervous tension.
BEAUTY	*Face:* blackheads/problem skin facial steam. *Body:* reviving bath infusion.

Lime flower
Tilia europaea

Formerly known as the linden tree, the lime tree and its flowers were traditionally used in Europe for treating colds and fevers as well as being a popular digestive and calming tea in France for many years. Tilleul, made with dried lime flowers, is a well-known after-dinner drink. Its gentle, relaxing properties are often employed to help parents cope with irritable children.

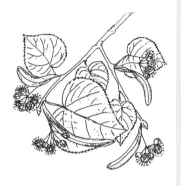

DESCRIPTION	A tall, deciduous tree with broad, oval, dark-green leaves, pale yellow, sweet-smelling flowers in spring and yellowish-green fruit.
PARTS USED	Flowers.
HEALTH	Its soothing and calming relaxant action is recommended for bronchitis, fever, high blood pressure, insomnia, nausea and vomiting, nervous tension, sciatica.
BEAUTY	*Face:* recommended for normal skin; deep cleansing mask for normal skin; blackheads/problem skin facial steam; lime flowers and avocado rich moisture cream. *Hair:* recommended for dry/sensitive hair; added shine and lustre; herbal tonic finishing rinse; lime flowers and yogurt flyaway hair formula. *Body:* relaxing bath infusion; skin softening milk bath. *Feet:* refreshing footbath.

Marigold (Pot)
Calendula officinalis

Due to its long flowering period, from early summer through to late autumn, this herb takes its name from the Latin *calendulae*, meaning 'throughout the months'. Marigold has long been used in Indian, Arabic and Greek medicine. Ancient Egyptians regarded it as a rejuvenating herb. Old French sources claimed that merely looking at the flowers for a few minutes each day would strengthen weak eyes. Garlands of the plant were once attached to door handles to keep evil, particularly contagion, out of the house. In the sixteenth century, marigold was a common garden plant valued by herbalists for comforting the heart and soothing the spirit. And the therapeutic values of the flowers in treating skin problems have long been known. For example, marigold poultices were used to heal and remove the scars of smallpox. In the American Civil War, the leaves were used to treat open wounds.

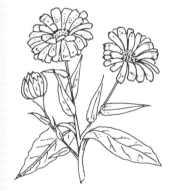

DESCRIPTION	An annual with hairy oblong leaves and large yellow or orange daisy-like flowers.
PARTS USED	Flowerheads, or flower petals alone.
HEALTH	A herbal astringent, antiseptic and anti-inflammatory. Recommended for acne and spots, athlete's foot, boils and sores, bruises, burns, conjunctivitis, cuts and wounds, eczema, haemorrhoids, herpes, psoriasis, sore throat, sprains, thrush, tonsillitis, toothache, varicose veins.
BEAUTY	*Face:* recommended for dry/sensitive skin; herbal moisturiser; sage and marigold astringent; peppermint and marigold compress for enlarged pores. *Eyes:* compress to soothe tired, sore and inflamed eyes. *Hair:* recommended for oily hair; anti-dandruff; added shine and lustre; colour enhancer for red hair. *Body:* bath infusion to relieve tired and aching muscles. *Hands:* herbal hand softening infusion; marigold and oatmeal hand cleanser; marigold hand cream. *Feet:* refreshing footbath; soothing footbath; marigold and lime foot lotion; peppermint foot balm.

Marshmallow
Althaea officinalis

An ancient food plant as well as a medicine, marshmallow is mentioned in the Bible and in Arabic and Chinese history as a valuable food for the poor and in famines. The ancient Greeks used it both as a medicine and a decoration for graves and it takes its name from the Greek word *altho*, 'to heal'. The marshmallow herb was the source of the confectionery of the same name, although the only similarity between today's spongy cubes and the original recipe is its sugar content.

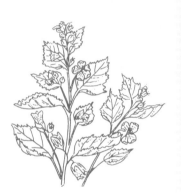

DESCRIPTION	A perennial herb with pale-green, stalked leaves, a thick, tapering, sweetish-tasting root and pale pink flowers in summer.
PARTS USED	Root, leaves.
HEALTH	The root of this herb produces a mucilage which soothes the stomach and gut. Recommended for acid stomach, acne and spots, bites and stings, boils and sores, colitis, coughs, diarrhoea, earache, indigestion, irritable bowel syndrome.
BEAUTY	*Face:* recommended for dry/sensitive skin; deep cleansing mask for dry/sensitive skin; dry/sensitive skin facial steam. *Hair:* recommended for dry/sensitive hair; herbal warm oil repair treatment. *Body:* relaxing bath infusion. *Hands:* herbal hand softening infusion; rough skin saver.

Meadowsweet
Filipendula ulmaria

A plant held sacred by the Druids. At weddings it was not only made into garlands for the bride and posies for the bridesmaids, but was also strewn along the route to the church and in the church itself. It was popular in Tudor times too with 'Queen Elizabeth of famous memory did more desire it than any other sweet herbe to strew her chambers withal'.

DESCRIPTION	A member of the rose family, it has rough, divided leaves which are dull green above and white and downy underneath. Creamy flowers appear on reddish stems in July and August. The scent of the flowers and leaves is entirely different.
PARTS USED	Flowers, leaves and root.
HEALTH	A herbal astringent and painkiller, meadowsweet is rich in salicylates, on which today's aspirin is based, although it doesn't cause irritation to the stomach lining often associated with the orthodox drug. Recommended for acid stomach, arthritis, diarrhoea, indigestion, rheumatism.
BEAUTY	*Body:* herbal all-over body tonic.

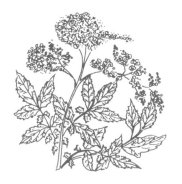

Milk thistle
Silybum marianum

According to the seventeenth-century diarist, John Evelyn, 'disarmed of its prickles and boiled, it is worthy of esteem and thought to be a great breeder of milk and proper diet for women who are nurses'. This association with lactation was probably due to the white veins on the leaves of this plant. According to folklore, when Mary was suckling Jesus a few drops of her milk fell on the leaf.

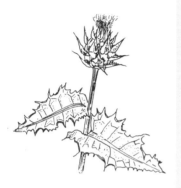

DESCRIPTION	A biennial with large, shiny leaves with white veins and sharp, yellowish prickles. Produces pink or white flowers from June to August.
PARTS USED	Seed.
HEALTH	A valuable tonic and protective agent for the liver. Recommended for a hangover and indigestion.

Myrrh
Commiphora molmol

A native plant of Africa and Arabia, myrrh has been widely used since ancient times in perfumes and incense. The modern name is derived from the Hebrew and Arabic word *mur* meaning 'bitter'. There are many Old Testament references to Myrrh and in the New Testament it is mentioned as one of the gifts brought by the Three Kings at the birth of Christ. In Greek mythology, Myrrh was turned into a tree by the gods to protect her from her father's anger at discovering she'd been tricked into incest. Her tears are said to be the resin which exudes from the bark. Later the herb was widely used as the herbalist's cleansing agent, countering poisons throughout the body.

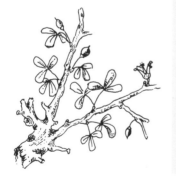

DESCRIPTION	A shrub with small, three-petalled leaves.
PARTS USED	Gum-resin which exudes from bark.
HEALTH	An antiseptic, astringent herb recommended for herpes, laryngitis, mouth ulcers, sore throat, tonsillitis, toothache.

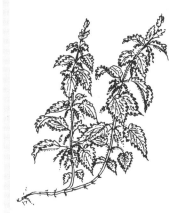

Nettle, common
Urtica dioica

The Romans used to beat their rheumatic joints with nettles and rub the leaves on their bodies to warm them up. The sting, which is caused by the formic acid in special hairs on the leaves, stimulates blood circulation, but drying or heating the leaves stops the stinging action.

DESCRIPTION   Heart-shaped leaves with normal and stinging hairs and flowers throughout summer.

Nettle, smaller
Urtica urens

DESCRIPTION   An annual which is a shorter version of the common nettle. And unlike the common nettle, the leaves are smooth and shiny except for the stinging hairs.

PARTS USED   Whole herb.

CAUTION   Fresh nettles should always be handled with gloves because of the sting carried in the leaves. Never use in their fresh state when applying to the body, without boiling beforehand to eliminate the sting.

HEALTH   Rich in minerals both varieties of this herb make an excellent tonic, a blood purifier, astringent and diuretic. Recommended for anaemia, athlete's foot, baldness, colds, eczema, haemorrhoids, rheumatism.

BEAUTY   *Face:* recommended for normal skin; deep cleansing mask for normal skin; deep cleansing facial steam. *Hair:* recommended for normal hair; added shine and lustre; improved growth; herbal tonic finishing rinse; herbal warm oil repair treatment. *Body:* herbal all-over tonic. *Feet:* refreshing footbath.

Oats
Avena sativa

Oats have probably been eaten, if not cultivated, since neolithic times. As a member of the grass family, which also include grains, this plant forms part of the staple diet of most of the world's population. Traditionally oats have been used as a nerve restorative and as a general tonic.

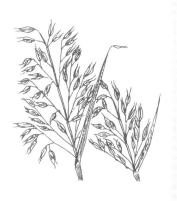

DESCRIPTION	A typical grain.
PARTS USED	Fresh whole plant or the dried grain.
HEALTH	The grain makes a nourishing food which benefits the nervous system. Recommended for depression, eczema, herpes, low blood pressure, nervous tension.
BEAUTY	*Face:* deep cleansing face pack; herbal exfoliator; elderflower and honey facial scrub. *Hands:* marigold and oatmeal hand cleanser; lady's mantle hand conditioner. *Body:* herbal body buffer; ivy anti-cellulite cream.

Parsley
Petroselinum crispum

The best-known and most commonly used herb in this country, parsley was thought of by the Greeks as sacred

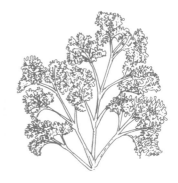

and was used to decorate tombs. It was also presented in the form of wreaths to the winning athletes who competed in the Isthmian Games. Only later in Roman times was it eaten as food. Culpeper recommended the herb for the stomach, kidney and menstrual problems.

DESCRIPTION	A biennial with divided leaves which are curled or flat depending on the type. It has a thick taproot, creamy-white clusters of flowers in summer followed by small, ribbed fruit. It also has a characteristic smell.
PARTS USED	Leaves, roots, seeds.
HEALTH	A diuretic and calming herb. Recommended for anaemia, arthritis, bad breath, rheumatism.
BEAUTY	*Face:* dry/sensitive skin facial steam; lavender anti-blemish night cream. *Mouth:* breath freshener. *Hair:* recommended for dry/sensitive hair; added shine and lustre; herbal warm oil repair treatment.

Peppermint
Mentha piperita

According to Greek mythology Minthe was a nymph loved by the god Pluto, who turned her into this scented herb to save her from his jealous wife. Peppermint became known as a symbol of hospitality to the Romans who used it to scent rooms where they would entertain guests. The Egyptians also used peppermint but it wasn't formally discovered in Britain until 1696. Its medicinal value was soon recognised and within 25 years of its description the herb was included in the London Pharmacopoeia. With its ability to interbreed so easily there are now over 30 species of mint.

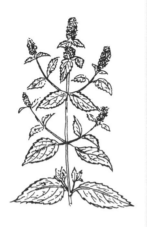

DESCRIPTION	A perennial with reddish-purple, square stems and shiny, oval, dark-green serrated leaves. Small purple flowers appear in summer. It has perhaps the strongest scent of all mint varieties.
PARTS USED	Whole herb.
CAUTION	Avoid prolonged use of inhalants of the oil. It can also irritate the mucus membranes and should not be given to children for longer than a week and shouldn't be given to babies in any form.
HEALTH	An anti-spasmodic, antiseptic herb which is also a mild relaxant. Recommended for athlete's foot, bad breath, bronchitis, catarrh, colds, dizziness, fever, flatulence, hangover, headache and migraine, indigestion, nausea and vomiting, sore throat, travel sickness.
BEAUTY	*Face:* recommended for normal skin; deep cleansing mask for normal skin; peppermint and marigold compress for enlarged pores. *Eyes:* compress to minimise dark circles. *Mouth:* breath freshener; peppermint and raspberry mouthwash; peppermint toothpaste. *Hair:* recommended for oily hair; anti-dandruff; minty-fresh hair rinse. *Body:* reviving bath infusion. *Feet:* refreshing footbath; soothing footbath; peppermint foot balm.

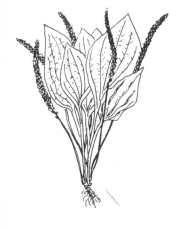

Plantain
Plantago major/plantago lanceolata

In an ancient Anglo-Saxon manual of medicinal preparations called the *Lacaunga* there is a song known as the 'lay
of the nine herbs'. One of these is given as waybread, the
old country name for plantain (plantago major). A piece of
root was once carried in the pocket to protect against
snakebites and plantain tea was recommended if suffering
from a venomous bite. Roman soldiers used to put the
leaves in their boots to prevent blisters. A closely related
species of the plant, *plantago lanceolata*, commonly known
as ribwort, was also a trusted plant for healing wounds.
Shakespeare mentions the herb in both *Romeo and Juliet*
and *Love's Labours Lost*.

DESCRIPTION	A perennial with a rosette of long, pointed oval, slightly hairy leaves. The greeny-white flowers grow on single, leafless stems that stand out above the foliage.
PARTS USED	Leaves.
HEALTH	An astringent and diuretic herb. *Plantago major* is recommended for bites and stings, boils and sores, conjunctivitis, diarrhoea, haemorrhoids. *Plantago lanceolata* is recommended for catarrh, cuts and wounds.
BEAUTY	*Plantago major* – *Face:* plantain problem skin lotion.

Rosemary
Rosmarinus officinalis

Rosemary, 'dew of the sea', so called because of its habit of
growing close to the sea, was a revered ceremonial herb,

symbolising remembrance, friendship and fidelity. In the Middle Ages it was believed to have mythical powers of protection against evil spirits and featured in both weddings and funerals. Placed under a bed it was said to guard against nightmares. It is still said that rosemary grows strongly in the kitchen gardens of households where the woman rules supreme. Rosemary has also been found to be extremely useful for improving mental concentration through its action of improving the flow of blood to the brain, and it is currently being looked at in relation to Alzheimer's disease.

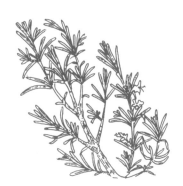

DESCRIPTION	A fragrant shrub with needle-like, bluey-green leaves and pink to pale-blue flowers which bloom April and May.
PARTS USED	Leaves.
HEALTH	An astringent herb, recommended for dizziness, headache and migraine, laryngitis, low blood pressure.
BEAUTY	*Face:* deep cleansing facial steam; rosemary skin booster. *Eyes:* rosemary puffy eyes lotion. *Hair:* recommended for oily hair; anti-dandruff; added shine and lustre; herbal tonic finishing rinse; colour enhancer for dark hair; rosemary pre-wash conditioner. *Body:* reviving bath infusion. *Feet:* refreshing footbath; deodorising footbath.

Sage
Salvia officinalis

Sage derives its name from the Latin *slavere*, 'to be in good health', and it has been considered a cure-all throughout history. 'How can a man grow old who has sage in his garden?' is the substance of an ancient proverb much quoted in China and Persia and parts of Europe. It was considered a sacred herb by the Greeks, who dedicated it to Zeus, and by the Romans who introduced it to Britain.

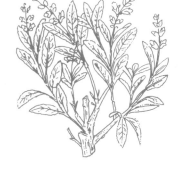

DESCRIPTION	A perennial shrub with wrinkled, oval leaves that can be reddish or green. Violet-blue, two-lipped flowers appear late summer.
PARTS USED	Leaves.
CAUTION	Sage should not be taken for medicinal purposes during pregnancy although small amounts used in cooking are perfectly safe.
HEALTH	A natural antibiotic and tonic which also aids digestion. Recommended for acne and spots, athlete's foot, colds, cuts and wounds, headache and migraine, laryngitis, menopause, mouth ulcers, sore throat, tonsillitis.
BEAUTY	*Face:* recommended for oily skin; deep cleansing mask for oily skin; oily skin facial steam; sage and marigold astringent. *Mouth:* tooth cleanser; apricot, banana and sage lip balm. *Hair:* recommended for dry/sensitive hair; anti-dandruff; added shine and lustre; colour enhancer for dark hair; colour enhancer for grey hair; sage and tea darkening lotion. *Body:* reviving bath infusion; bath infusion to relieve tired and aching muscles. *Feet:* refreshing footbath; deodorising footbath.

St John's wort
Hypericum perforatum

Wort is an Anglo-Saxon word meaning 'a medicinal herb'. Some believe it got its name because of its traditional association with St John the Baptist. As its yellow flowers turn red when crushed, this red colour came to represent his blood. Others say it was so called because it was used by the Knights of the Order of St John to heal wounds suffered during the Crusades. When crushed this herb gives a strong balsamic aroma like incense and the smell was believed to drive evil away. Medicinally the herb is highly regarded for the soothing and healing properties of the red oil obtained from the flowers and the leaves.

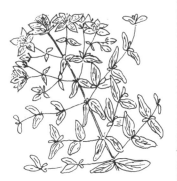

DESCRIPTION	A perennial with woody stems, it has oval-shaped small, thin, veined leaves covered in translucent dots that contain an essential oil which is also found in the small, golden-yellow flowers.
PARTS USED	Flowering herb.
CAUTION	Due to its photosensitivity, sunbathing or long exposure to bright sunlight should be avoided when taking St John's wort.
HEALTH	An astringent which is also soothing to the nervous system. Recommended for cuts and wounds, depression, earache, haemorrhoids, herpes, menopause, psoriasis, sciatica, sprains.
BEAUTY	*Face:* recommended for normal skin; herbal moisturiser. *Hair:* colour enhancer for blonde/fair hair.

Slippery elm
Ulmus fulva

The common name of this herb comes from the feel of its moistened inner bark. The North American Indians used it as a treatment for diarrhoea because of the soothing and protective mucilage it provides. Once it became known in Europe, it was also used as a healing poultice.

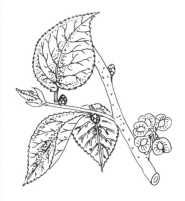

DESCRIPTION   A tree with rough bark and oval, serrated leaves and tiny flowers which grow in clusters.

PARTS USED   Inner bark.

HEALTH   A healing, nutritious herb with a gentle action effective in soothing irritated tissue. Recommended for acid stomach, acne and spots, boils and sores, colitis, diarrhoea, indigestion.

Thyme
Garden thyme/thymus vulgaris; *Wild thyme/thymus serpyllum*

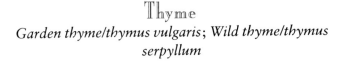

The word 'thymus' derives from the Greek word *thymon* meaning 'courage', and the herb has been linked to this virtue throughout the ages. Roman soldiers bathed in thyme water before battle. In the Middle Ages, women embroidered a sprig of thyme into the clothes of knights before they went off to fight in the Crusades. Thyme was also carried by judges and kings to protect them from disease in public. The Egyptians developed the powerful antiseptic and preservative properties of the herb and used it for embalming. It is also an excellent bee plant and traditionally was always planted close to hives.

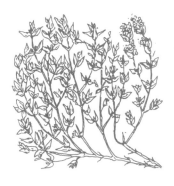

DESCRIPTION Both plants are perennial, low aromatic shrubs. Common thyme has pink flowers and short, pointed leaves. Wild thyme has reddish-purple flowers and small, oval leaves.

PARTS USED Whole herb.

HEALTH Both varieties contain similar properties and act as an astringent and expectorant and have a calming effect on the digestive tract. Recommended for acne and spots, asthma, bronchitis, catarrh, colds, coughs, cystitis, diarrhoea, hangover, laryngitis, nausea and vomiting, nervous tension, sore throat, thrush, tonsillitis.

BEAUTY *Hair:* recommended for improved growth. *Body:* reviving bath infusion. *Feet:* refreshing footbath; soothing footbath.

Valerian
Valeriana officinalis

This ancient medicinal herb, whose name comes from the Latin *valere*, 'to be in health', has been valued throughout history. Hippocrates recommended valerian in the fourth century BC and it was used in the recipes for leeching used by Anglo-Saxon herbalists. Valerian was supposed to inspire love, and if a girl wore the herb she would never lack lovers. It is also known as 'All Heal' because of the high esteem in which it was held in the Middle Ages when it was widely grown in monastery gardens and used as a spice and as a perfume. The distinctive smell of the herb does not come from the fresh plant itself but from the dried root which is used to add a musky tone to perfume. It is said that cats and rats are attracted by the smell of valerian and that the Pied Piper of Hamelin made the rats follow him by putting the herb in his pocket. During the Second World War, people suffering with shell shock and nervous stress were treated with valerian.

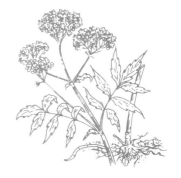

DESCRIPTION	A perennial with a short rhizome and thin roots and a rosette of divided leaves. Its flowers are white tinged with pink and bloom in midsummer.
PARTS USED	Rhizome and/or roots.
CAUTION	Avoid large doses over a prolonged period of time. Valerian can also increase the effect of certain sleeping pills and should not be used if taking sleeping pills unless under professional guidance.
HEALTH	A general sedative and relaxant. Recommended for arthritis, colitis, diarrhoea, headache and migraine, high blood pressure, insomnia, irritable bowel syndrome, menopause, nervous tension, painful periods, premenstrual tension, psoriasis, rheumatism, sciatica, toothache.
BEAUTY	*Face:* blackheads/problem skin facial steam. *Body:* relaxing bath infusion.

Vervain
Verbena officinalis

Vervain has been known and used in Europe for many centuries. Its name comes from the Celtic *ferfaen*, meaning 'to drive away a stone', and refers to its use in bladder infections. It was also regarded as an aphrodisiac. In ancient Greece, Hippocrates, the 'father of medicine', applied vervain to wounds and prescribed its use in fevers and nervous disorders. Legend has it that vervain was originally found on Mount Calvary and used to staunch the wounds of Christ, which is possibly why, medicinally, it was thought to cure every ill. In the Middle Ages magicians used it for casting spells or adding to potions, particularly love potions. It was used to foretell the future and protect houses against wicked spirits, and it was worn around the neck as a general good luck charm.

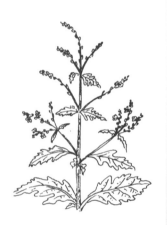

DESCRIPTION   A perennial with a branched squarish stem, with lobed leaves and tiny blue flowers arranged in long, slender spikes at the top of the stalks which bloom from July to September.

PARTS USED   Leaves.

HEALTH   A natural relaxant and anti-spasmodic herb. Recommended for conjunctivitis, depression, fever, headache and migraine, nervous tension, psoriasis.

BEAUTY   *Body:* relaxing bath infusion.

Witch hazel
Hamamelis virginiana

Witch hazel has a long history of use among the American Indians, who used its twigs for water divining and its leaves and bark as an astringent and tonic.

DESCRIPTION   Perennial shrub with smooth bark, toothed oval leaves and yellow flowers followed by small black nuts containing white seeds.

PARTS USED   Leaves, bark, twigs. Distilled witch hazel, which is made from the young flower-

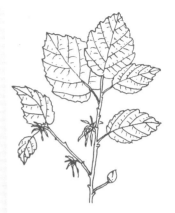

bearing twigs, can be bought from all good chemists.

CAUTION Tincture of witch hazel (not to be confused with distilled witch hazel) is a strong astringent. Handle with care as it stains badly.

HEALTH A natural astringent, it also helps staunch bleeding. Recommended for bites and stings, bruises, burns, conjunctivitis, cuts and wounds, haemorrhoids, hay fever, sprains, varicose veins.

BEAUTY *Face:* sage and marigold astringent. *Mouth:* witch hazel mouthwash. *Hair:* recommended for oily hair; anti-dandruff. *Body:* herbal all-over body tonic.

Yarrow
Achillea millefolium

The Latin name for yarrow is said to be derived from the fact that the Greek hero Achilles used the herb to treat soldiers' wounds. Long considered sacred, yarrow stems were used by the Druids to foretell the weather, while in China yarrow stems were used to foretell the future. The *I Ching* or *Book of Changes* was also known as the *Yarrow Stalk Oracle*.

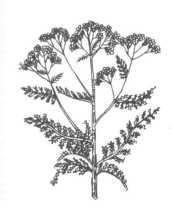

DESCRIPTION A perennial, creeping herb. The stem is angular with a profusion of long, greygreen leaves that look like fern fronds. Small, white or pink-tinged flowers with yellow centres grow in loose clusters at the top of the plant in summer.

PARTS USED The flowering herb.

CAUTION Essentially a very safe herb but in rare cases

excessive doses can cause dizziness and vertigo or an allergic skin reaction.

HEALTH A natural antiseptic and good digestive herb. Recommended for acid stomach, acne and spots, bronchitis, colds, coughs, cuts and wounds, fever, haemorrhoids, hangover, hay fever, high blood pressure, laryngitis, nausea and vomiting, psoriasis.

BEAUTY *Face:* recommended for oily skin; deep cleansing mask for oily skin; oily skin facial steam. *Hair:* recommended for oily hair; anti-dandruff. *Hands:* herbal hand softening infusion. *Body:* bath infusion to relieve tired and aching muscles.

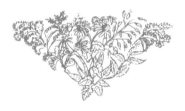

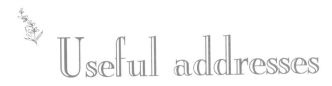

Useful addresses

British Herbal Medicine Association
Field House, Lyle Hole Lane, Redhill, Avon BS18 7TB.
Tel: 0934 862994

Iden Croft Herbs
Frittenden Road, Staplehurst, Kent TN12 0DH.
Tel: 0580 891432

The Natural Medicines Society
Edith Lewis House, Ilkeston, Derbyshire DE7 8EJ.
Tel: 0602 329454

The Herb Society
PO Box 599, London SW11 4RW.

The National Institute of Medical Herbalists
9 Palace Gate, Exeter, Devon EX1 1JA.
Tel: 0392 426022

Dried herb suppliers

All offer a mail order service

G Baldwin & Co
173 Walworth Road, London SE17 1RW.
Tel: 071 703 5550

Brome & Schimmer Ltd
Unit 42, Romsey Industrial Estate, Great Bridge Road,
   Romsey, Hampshire SO51 0HR.
Tel: 0794 515595

Culpeper Ltd (Head Office)
Hadstock Road, Linton, Cambridgeshire CB1 6NJ.
Tel: 0223 894054

The Herbal Apothecary
103 The High Street, Syston, Leicestershire LE7 8GQ.
Tel: 0533 602690

Neal's Yard Remedies
5 Golden Cross, Corn Market Street, Oxford OX1 3EU.
Tel: 0865 245436

Phyto Products Ltd
3 Kings Mill Way, Hermitage Lane, Mansfield,
   Nottinghamshire NG18 5ER.
Tel: 0623 644334

Potter's Herbal Supplies Ltd
Leyland Mill Lane, Wigan, Lancashire WN1 2SB.
Tel: 0942 34761

Training courses in herbal medicine

The School of Phytotherapy (Herbal Medicine)
Bucksteep Manor, Bodle Street Green, Hailsham,
   East Sussex BN27 4RJ.
Tel: 0323 833812/4

Beauty

Cosmetics To Go
Freepost, Poole, Dorset BH15 1BR.
For the Cosmetics To Go latest brochure call freephone:
   0800 373 366

Montagne Jeunesse
The Business Village, Broomhill Road, London SW18 4JQ
Tel: 081 877 3227

Recommended reading

The A–Z of Modern Herbalism, Simon Mills, Thorsons 1989.

Aromatherapy: The Encyclopaedia of Plants and Oils and How they Help You, Daniele Ryman, Piatkus 1991.

The Complete Book of Herbs, Lesley Bremness, Dorling Kindersley 1988.

The Complete New Herbal, Richard Mabey (consultant editor), Elm Tree Books UK 1988.

The Country Diary Herbal, Sarah Hollis, Webb & Bower 1990.

A Country Herbal, Lesley Gordon, Webb & Bower 1980.

Culpeper's Colour Herbal, David Potterton, W. Foulsham & Co 1983.

The Encyclopaedia of Herbs and Herbalism, Malcolm Stuart, Orbis 1987.

The Herb Society's Complete Medicinal Herbal, Penelope Ody, Dorling Kindersley 1993.

Herbs for Common Ailments, Anne McIntyre, Gaia 1992.

The Herbal for Mother and Child, Anne McIntyre, Element 1992.

The Illustrated Herbal, Philippa Back, Hamlyn 1987.

Natural Beauty: The Practical Guide to Wildflower Cosmetics, Roy Genders, Webb & Bower 1988.

The Natural Beauty Book, Anita Guyton, Thorsons 1991.

Natural Health Handbook, Dr Anthony Campbell, New Burlington Books 1991.

The Natural Pharmacy, Miriam Polunin and Christopher Robbins, Dorling Kindersley 1992.

Index

Page numbers in bold refer to main herb entries in chapter 5 The A–Z of Herbs.
Page numbers in italics refer to ailments found in chapter 4 Herbs for Health.